a LANGE medical book

CU[
Prac
In Primary Care
2004

Laura Guerrero
205 Barkley Ave.
Clifton, NJ 07011-3139

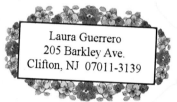

Ralph Gonzales, MD, MSPH

Associate Professor
Division of General Internal Medicine
Department of Medicine
University of California, San Francisco
San Francisco, California

Jean S. Kutner, MD, MSPH

Associate Professor and Interim Chief
Division of General Internal Medicine
Department of Medicine
University of Colorado Health Sciences Center
Denver, Colorado

Lange Medical Books/McGraw-Hill
Medical Publishing Division

New York   Chicago   San Francisco   Lisbon   London
Madrid   Mexico City   Milan   New Delhi   San Juan   Seoul
Singapore   Sydney   Toronto

The **McGraw·Hill** Companies

CURRENT Practice Guidelines in Primary Care, 2004

Copyright © 2004, 2003, 2002, 2000, by The **McGraw-Hill Companies,** Inc.
All rights reserved. Printed in the United States of America. Except as
permitted under the United States Copyright Act of 1976, no part of this
publication may be reproduced or distributed in any form or by any means, or
stored in a data base or retrieval system, without the prior written permission
of the publisher.

1 2 3 4 5 6 7 8 9 0 DOC/DOC 0 9 8 7 6 5 4

ISBN: 0-07-143361-9
ISSN: 1528-1612

Notice

Medicine is an ever-changing science. As new research and clinical experience broaden our knowledge, changes in treatment and drug therapy are
required. The authors and the publisher of this work have checked with
sources believed to be reliable in their efforts to provide information that
is complete and generally in accord with the standards accepted at the time
of publication. However, in view of the possibility of human error or
changes in medical sciences, neither the authors nor the publisher nor any
other party who has been involved in the preparation or publication of this
work warrants that the information contained herein is in every respect
accurate or complete, and they disclaim all responsibility for any errors or
omissions or for the results obtained from use of the information contained in this work. Readers are encouraged to confirm the information
contained herein with other sources. For example and in particular, readers are advised to check the product information sheet included in the
package of each drug they plan to administer to be certain that the information contained in this work is accurate and that changes have not been
made in the recommended dose or in the contraindications for administration. This recommendation is of particular importance in connection with
new or infrequently used drugs.

This book was set in Times New Roman by Silverchair Science + Communications.
The editor was Shelley Reinhardt.
The production supervisor was Phil Galea.
RR Donnelley was the printer and binder.
This book is printed on acid-free paper.

Contents

A Report Card on U.S. Health Care Delivery   *Inside Front Cover*
Preface   *vii*
Abbreviations   *Inside Back Cover*

1. DISEASE SCREENING

Alcohol Abuse & Dependence 2
√ Anemia 4
Cancer
    Bladder 5
√   Breast 6
√   Cervical 10
√   Colorectal 14
    Endometrial 18
    Gastric 19
√   Liver 20
√   Lung 21
    Oral 22
    Ovarian 23
    Pancreatic 25
√   Prostate 26
    Skin 28
    Testicular 29
    Thyroid 30
√ Carotid Artery Stenosis 31
Child Abuse & Neglect 33
√ Chlamydial Infection 34
Cholesterol & Lipid Disorders
    Children 35
    Adults 36
√ Dementia 38
Depression 39
√ Diabetes Mellitus
√   Gestational 41
√   Type 2 42

"√" denotes major 2004 updates.

Domestic Violence & Abuse 43
√ Falls in the Elderly 44
Hearing Impairment 45
√ Hepatitis B Virus 47
√ Hepatitis C Virus 48
HCV Infection Testing Algorithm 49
Human Immunodeficiency Virus 50
√ Hypertension
√   Children & Adolescents 52
√   Adults 53
Elderly 54
Lead Poisoning 55
Obesity 57
√ Osteoporosis 58
Osteoporosis Screening Algorithm 59
Risk Factors 60
Secondary Osteoporosis 61
Scoliosis 62
Syphilis 63
Thyroid Disease 64
√ Tuberculosis 66
Visual Impairment, Glaucoma, & Cataracts 68

2. DISEASE PREVENTION

√ Breast Cancer 72
√ Diabetes, Type 2 74
Endocarditis 75
√ Falls in the Elderly 76
√ Hypertension 77
√   Hypertension Prevention Algorithm 78
√ Myocardial Infarction 79
√ Osteoporosis 81
Osteoporosis Prevention Algorithm 83
√ Stroke 84
Vaccines for Children 86
Vaccines for Adults 89

"√" denotes major 2004 updates.

3. DISEASE MANAGEMENT

Allergic Rhinitis
    Diagnosis & Management 94
Arthritis: Hip & Knee
    Pharmacological Management 96
    Exercise Prescription 98
Asthma
    Severity Classification 99
    Treatment 101
√ Atopic Dermatitis
    Evaluation & Management 106
√ Atrial Fibrillation
    Evaluation & Management 109
√ Carotid Artery Stenosis
    Evaluation & Management 111
Cataracts in Adults
    Evaluation & Management 112
Chest Pain (Non-Traumatic)
    Actions in Response to Important Historical Elements 114
    Actions in Response to Important Physical Examination
        Findings 116
Depression
    Management 118
Diabetes Mellitus
√   Management of Hyperglycemia 119
√   Prevention & Treatment of Diabetic Complications 120
Heart Failure 123
√ Hormone Replacement Therapy
    Risks & Benefits 124
√ Hypertension
    Initiating Treatment 127
    Lifestyle Modifications 128
    Recommended Medications for Compelling Indications 129
    Causes of Resistant Hypertension 130
Lipid & Cholesterol Management 131
√ Low Back Pain, Acute
    Initial Evaluation 132
    Treatment 133
    Evaluation of Slow-To-Recover Patient 134

"√" denotes major 2004 updates.

Persistent Sciatica 135
Red Flags for Potentially Serious Conditions 136
Obesity Management
Adults 138
Children 139
√ Osteoporosis Management 140
√ PAP Smear Abnormalities
Management & Follow-Up 141
Perioperative Cardiovascular Evaluation 142
Pneumonia (Community-Acquired) 144
Upper Respiratory Tract Infections
Cough Illness (Bronchitis) 145
Acute Sore Throat (Pharyngitis) 146
Acute Nasal and Sinus Congestion (Sinusitis) 147
Urinary Tract Infections in Women
Diagnosis & Management 148
Notes & Tables 149

4. APPENDICES

Appendix I: Screening Instruments
Alcohol Abuse (CAGE, AUDIT) 152
Cognitive Impairment (MMSE) 155
Depression 157
Beck Depression Inventory (Short Form) 158
Geriatric Depression Scale 159
Appendix II: Functional Assessment Screening in the Elderly 161
Appendix III: 95th Percentile of Blood Pressure for Boys and Girls
Boys 164
Girls 165
Appendix IV: Body Mass Index Conversion Table 166
Appendix V: Cardiac Risk-Framingham Study
Men 167
Women 168
√ Appendix VI: Professional Societies & Governmental Agencies
Acronyms & Internet Sites 169
Appendix VII: References 171

Index 173

"√" denotes major 2004 updates.

Preface

Current Practice Guidelines in Primary Care 2004 is intended for primary care clinicians. These include not only residents and practicing physicians in the specialties of family medicine, internal medicine, pediatrics, and obstetrics and gynecology but also medical and nursing students during their ambulatory care rotations, registered nurses, nurse practitioners, and physician assistants. Its purpose is to make *screening, primary prevention*, and *management* recommendations readily accessible and available for clinical decision making. The recommendations included are issued regularly by governmental agencies, expert panels, medical specialty organizations, and other professional and scientific organizations.

Current Practice Guidelines in Primary Care 2004 is essential for the busy clinician. New recommendations are continually being published by organizations that express different positions on the same topics, and current guidelines require revision as new evidence from clinical and outcomes research emerges. The intent of this guide is both to help clinicians select the most appropriate clinical preventive services and interventions for a given situation and to provide clinicians with quick access to the latest information.

Current Practice Guidelines in Primary Care 2004 has been updated using PubMed searches limited to articles published in English between 1/1/02 to 10/20/03 and "practice guideline" publication type, as well as via the Web sites of major professional societies, the Agency for Healthcare Research and Quality Guidelines Clearinghouse, and the U.S. Preventive Services Task Force. This updating strategy led to substantial modification of many guidelines (look for "√" in the Contents). New material has been added addressing prevention of type 2 diabetes and hypertension and screening for and prevention of falls in the elderly.

Ralph Gonzales, MD, MSPH
Associate Professor of Medicine
University of California, San Francisco
San Francisco, California

Jean S. Kutner, MD, MSPH
Associate Professor of Medicine and Interim Chief
University of Colorado Health Sciences Center
Denver, Colorado

January 2004

1
Disease Screening

ALCOHOL ABUSE & DEPENDENCE

Disease Screening	Organization	Date	Population	Recommendations	Comments	Source
Alcohol Abuse & Dependence	GAPS AAP Bright Futures	1997 1995	Adolescents	Ask all adolescents annually about their use of alcohol. Parents should also routinely receive instructions on monitoring their adolescent's social and recreational activities for use of alcohol.[a]	The finding of alcohol use or abuse should provoke an assessment of other conditions that co-vary with alcohol abuse, such as cigarette smoking, sexual activity, and mood disorders. Guidelines on treatment of alcohol abuse in adolescence have been published. (J Am Acad Child Adolesc Psychiatry 1998;37:122)	Arch Pediatr Adolesc Med 1997;151:123 Pediatrics 1995;95:439
	USPSTF	1996	Adolescents and adults	Screen all adolescents and adults using relevant history or a standardized screening instrument (see Appendix 1 for CAGE and AUDIT instruments).	A recent systematic review concluded that the Alcohol Use Disorders Identification Test (AUDIT) was most effective in identifying subjects with at-risk, hazardous, or harmful drinking (sensitivity, 51%–79%; specificity, 78%–96%); while the CAGE questions proved superior for detecting alcohol abuse and dependence (sensitivity, 43%–94%; specificity 70%–97%). (Arch Intern Med 2000;160:1977) Screening coupled with brief physician advice is cost-effective. (Med Care 2000;38:7)	

ALCOHOL ABUSE & DEPENDENCE

Disease Screening	Organization	Date	Population	Recommendations	Comments	Source
Alcohol Abuse & Dependence (continued)	NIAAA	2002	College students	Screen all students on National Alcohol Screening Day.[b]	1,400 college students between the ages of 18 and 24 die each year from alcohol-related injuries. (J Studies Alcohol 2002;63:136) Targeting only those with identified problems misses students who drink heavily or misuse alcohol occasionally. Nondependent, high-risk drinkers account for majority of alcohol-related deaths & damage.	http://www.collegedrinkingprevention.gov/Reports/TaskForce/CallToAction_01.aspx
	AAP ACOG	1997	Pregnant women	Counsel all pregnant women regarding the maternal health and fetal effects of alcohol during pregnancy.		AAP and ACOG: Guidelines for Perinatal Care, 4th ed. ACOG, 1997

[a]The AAP also acknowledges the importance of family attitudes toward alcohol and recommends that clinicians urge parents to use alcohol safely and in moderation, to restrict children from family alcohol supplies, and to recognize the influence their own drinking patterns can have on their children and parenting.
[b]National Alcohol Screening Day is April 8, 2004; sponsored by the National Institute on Alcohol Abuse and Alcoholism and other organizations (http://mentalhealthscreening.org/alcohol.htm).

ANEMIA

Disease Screening	Organization	Date	Population	Recommendations	Comments	Source
Anemia, Iron-Deficient	AAP	1993	Neonates	Universal hematocrit screening is not recommended.		Pediatrics 1993;92:474
	AAFP USPSTF	2002 1996	Infants aged 6–12 months	Perform selective, single hemoglobin or hematocrit screening for high-risk infants. [a]		
	CDC	1998	Infants and preschool children at high risk (migrants, refugees, and low income)	Screen all children for anemia between 9 and 12 months, 6 months later, and annually from 2 to 5 years.		MMWR 1998;47: RR-3
			Adolescent and adult women	Screen all nonpregnant women beginning in adolescence every 5–10 years until menopause.		
	CDC USPSTF	1998 1996	Pregnant women	Screen all women with hemoglobin or hematocrit at first prenatal visit.	When acute stress or inflammatory disorders are not present, a serum ferritin level is the most accurate test for evaluating iron deficiency anemia. Among women of childbearing age, a cut-off of 15 mg/dL has sensitivity of 75%, specificity of 98%. (Br J Haematol 1993;85:787)	

[a] Includes infants living in poverty, blacks, Native Americans and Alaska Natives, immigrants from developing countries, preterm and low birthweight infants, and infants whose principal dietary intake is unfortified cow's milk.

CANCER, BLADDER					
Disease Screening	Organization	Date	Population	Recommendations	Comments	Source

Disease Screening	Organization	Date	Population	Recommendations	Comments	Source
Cancer, Bladder	NCI	2003	Asymptomatic persons[a]	There is insufficient evidence to determine whether a decrease in mortality occurs with screening of any type.		http://www.cancer.gov/cancer_information/testing
	AAFP USPSTF CTF	2002 1996 1994	Asymptomatic persons[a]	Routine screening with microscopic urinalysis, urine dipstick, or urine cytology is *not* recommended.	Dipstick testing is sensitive and specific for hematuria, but hematuria is not specific for bladder cancer.	www.aafp.org/exam.xml

[a]Increased risk: exposure to azodyes, aromatic amines, and 4-aminobiphenyl; employment in the leather, tire, or rubber industries; and cigarette smoking (OR/RR 1.5–7.0). Persons working in high-risk professions may be eligible for screening at the worksite, although the benefit of this has not been determined. People who smoke should be advised that smoking significantly increases the risk for bladder cancer, and all smokers should be routinely counseled to quit smoking. A high index of suspicion should be maintained in anyone with a history of smoking or exposure to another risk factor.

				CANCER, BREAST		
Disease Screening	Organization	Date	Population[a]	Recommendations[b]	Comments	Source
Cancer, Breast	ASCO	2003	Women aged ≥ 20 years	Monthly BSE		www.asco.org
	ACS CTF	2001	Women aged ≥ 20 years	BSE: Women should report any breast change promptly to their health care provider. Women should be told about the benefits and limitations of BSE. It is acceptable for women to choose not to do BSE or to do it occasionally.	The value of BSE in reducing breast cancer mortality remains unproved. (Br J Cancer 1993;68:208)	www.cancer.org www.ctfphc.org
	ACS ASCO ACOG AMA	2003 2003 2002 2002	Women aged 20–39 years	CBE every 3 years		www.cancer.org www.asco.org www.acog.org www.ama-assn.org
	ACS ASCO ACOG AMA ACR	2003 2003 2002 2002 2002	Women aged ≥40 years	Mammography and CBE yearly	The CBE should be conducted close in time to the scheduled mammogram. A normal mammogram in the presence of a palpable mass does not rule out breast cancer.	www.cancer.org www.asco.org www.acog.org www.ama-assn.org www.acr.org CA Cancer J Clin 2002;52:8–22

Disease Screening	**Organization**	**Date**	**Population[a]**	**Recommendations[b]**	**Comments**	**Source**
Cancer, Breast (continued)	USPSTF	2002	Women aged ≥ 40 years	Mammography, with or without CBE, every 1–2 years	Thirty percent of all women screened annually at ages 40–49 will have at least 1 false-positive mammogram. (J Natl Cancer Inst 1997;22:139)	www.ahrq.gov/clinic/3rduspstf/breastcancer
	AAFP NCI	2002 2002	Women aged ≥ 40 years	Mammography every 1–2 years	Extending screening to include ages 40–49 improves life expectancy by 2.5 days at a cost of $676 per woman. Incremental cost-effectiveness is $105,000 per year of life saved. (Ann Intern Med 1997;127:955) RCTs consistently demonstrate no benefit from screening in the first 5–7 years after study entry. At 10–12 years, benefit is uncertain. [J Natl Cancer Inst 1993;85(20):1644] Number needed to screen to save 1 life = 2,500. [J Natl Cancer Inst 1997;89(14):1015] Risk-based recommendations may assist in counseling. [J Clin Oncol 1998;16(9):3105]	http://cancernet.nci.nih.gov http://www.cancer.gov/cancer_information www.aafp.org/exam.xml
	CTF	2001	Women aged 40–49 years	Counsel about risks/benefits of mammography and CBE.		CMAJ 2001;164(4):469–476 www.ctfphc.org

Disease Screening	Organization	Date	Population[a]	Recommendations[b]	Comments	Source
CANCER, BREAST						
Cancer, Breast (continued)	ACP AMA	1991 1989	Women aged 50–69 years	Mammography and CBE yearly	Screening women aged 50–69 years improves life expectancy by 12 days at a cost of $704 per woman, with a cost-effectiveness ratio of $21,400 per year of life saved. (Am Intern Med 1997;127:955)	www.acponline.org www.ama-assn.org JAMA 1989;261(17):2535
	CTF ACPM	1998 1996	Women aged 50–69 years	Mammography and CBE every 1–2 years		www.ctfphc.org www.acpm.org/breast.htm
	AGS ACPM	1999 1996	Women aged ≥ 70 years	Mammography and CBE every 1–2 years, with no upper age limit for women with an estimated life expectancy of ≥ 4 years. AGS recommends, in addition, monthly BSE.	Currently available data for women aged > 70 are inadequate to judge the effectiveness of screening. [J Natl Cancer Inst 1993;85(20):1644] Screening mammography in frail older women frequently necessitates work-up that offers no benefit. Encouraging individualized decisions may allow screening to be targeted to older women for whom the potential benefit outweighs the potential burdens. (J Gen Intern Med 2001;16:779–784)	www.americangeriatrics.org www.acpm.org/breast.htm

Disease Screening	Organization	Date	Population[a]	Recommendations[b]	Comments	Source
Cancer, Breast (continued)	ASCO	2000	Women	Present data are insufficient to recommend use of tumor markers (CA15-3, CEA) for screening for breast cancer.		J Clin Oncol 2001;19:1865–1878

[a]Women with a mother and sister with breast cancer have an RR > 4.0 of developing breast cancer. It is likely that < 10% of all breast cancer in Western countries is attributable to genetic predisposition. It has been estimated that 25% of breast cancers diagnosed before age 40 years are attributable to *BRCA1* mutations. Studies have not addressed when to begin breast cancer screening, and at what intervals, for women at high risk of breast cancer because of genetic predisposition. (Annu Rev Public Health 1996;17:47) Women known to be at increased risk may benefit from earlier initiation of mammogram and/or the addition of breast ultrasound or MRI. (ACS)

[b]Debate about the value of screening mammograms was triggered by a Cochrane review published on October 20, 2001 (Lancet 2001;358:1340–1342). This review cited a number of methodologic and analytic flaws in the large long-term mammography trials. The USPSTF and NCI concluded that the flaws were problematic but unlikely to negate the consistent and significant mortality reductions observed in the trials.

Summary of current evidence: NEJM 2003;348:1672–1680.

Disease Screening	Organization	Date	Population	Recommendations[a,c,d]	Comments	Source
CANCER, CERVICAL						
Cancer, Cervical	ACOG ACS	2003 2002	Women within 3 years after first sexual intercourse or by age 21, whichever comes first[e]	Annual Pap smear until age 30 (every 2 years if liquid-based Pap test, ACS) At age ≥ 30, if 3 consecutive normal results, may screen every 2–3 years. If negative on *both* Pap smear and HPV DNA test, rescreen with combined tests every 3 years. (ACOG)	Cervical cancer is causally related to infection with HPV. (http://odp.od.nih.gov/consensus/) 20%–60% reduction in cervical cancer mortality rates after implementation of screening programs. [Ann Intern Med 1990;113(3):214] As compared with annual screening for 3 years, screening performed once every 3 years after the last negative test in women aged 30–64 years who have had ≥ 3 consecutive negative Pap smears is associated with an average excess risk of approximately 3 in 100,000. (NEJM 2003;349:1501–1509)	www.acog.org www.cancer.org
	ASCO	2003	Women within 3 years after first sexual intercourse or by age 21, whichever comes first[e]	Pap smear at least every 2–3 years	Lead time from precancerous lesions to invasive cancer is 8–9 years. (Clinician's Handbook of Preventive Services. U.S. Government Printing Office, 1994) Single screening Pap test for detecting CIN grades I and II has sensitivity 14%–99%, specificity 24%–96%. (Am J Epidemiol 1995;141:680) The rate of false-negative results may be as high as 50%. An estimated 1/2 to 2/3 of false-negative results are caused by inadequate specimen collection and by misinterpreting or not observing abnormal cells. Recent studies have provided strong evidence that HPV DNA testing may have a strong role in identifying precancerous lesions and managing minor Pap abnormalities. (Ann Intern Med 2000;133:1021–1024)	www.asco.org

	CANCER, CERVICAL				
Disease Screening	**Organization**	**Date**	**Population**	**Recommendations**[a,c,d]	**Comments**	**Source**
Cancer, Cervical (continued)	Bright Futures GAPS	2002 1994	Women who are or have been sexually active[b]	Pap smear (with endocervical brush and spatula) and pelvic exam every year; if >3 consecutive normal exams, may perform less frequently at physician discretion.		www.brightfutures. org

Disease Screening	Organization	Date	Population	Recommendations[a,c,d]	Comments	Source
CANCER, CERVICAL						
Cancer, Cervical (continued)	NCI	2002	Women who are or have been sexually active OR Women aged > 18 years[b]	Regular screening with Pap smear decreases mortality. The upper age limit at which screening ceases to be effective is unknown.		http://cancernet.nci.nih.gov
	USPSTF AAFP ACP	2003 2002 1990	Women who have ever had sex and have a cervix[b,e]	Pap smear at least every 3 years	USPSTF notes that most of the benefit can be obtained by beginning screening within 3 years of onset of sexual activity or age 21.	www.aafp.org/exam. xml Ann Intern Med 1990;113(3):214
	ACPM CTF	1996 1994	Women who have ever had sex[b,e]	Pap smear every year for 2 years; if 2 normal annual smears, lengthen screening interval to 3 years at physician discretion.		www.acpm.org/ cervical.htm

CANCER, CERVICAL						
Disease Screening	Organization	Date	Population	Recommendations[a,c,d]	Comments	Source
Cancer, Cervical (continued)	ASCO	2003	Women aged > 65 years (aged > 70 years, ACS)	Discontinue screening if: regular screening, 2 satisfactory smears, no abnormal smears within previous 10 years, and not otherwise at high risk for cervical cancer. If no previous screening, 3 normal smears before discontinuation.	28%–64% of women aged > 65 have never had a Pap smear or have not had one done within 3 years. (Mt Sinai J Med 1985;52:284) In one study, women 65 years of age and older were 21% less likely than younger women to ever have had a Pap test and 33% less likely to have had a Pap test recently. Physician recommendation is the strongest predictor of whether a woman receives a Pap test. (Ann Intern Med 2000;133:1021–1024)	www.asco.org www.cancer.org www.acpm.org/ cervical.htm
	USPSTF	2003				
	ACS	2002				
	ACPM	1996				
	AGS	2000	Women aged > 65 years	Pap smear every 1–3 years until age 70. If no or insufficient prior Pap smears, 2 annual smears before discontinuation.	Beyond age 70, there is little evidence for or against screening women who have been regularly screened in previous years. Individual circumstances such as the patient's life expectancy, ability to undergo treatment if cancer is detected, and ability to cooperate with and tolerate the Pap smear procedure may obviate the need for cervical cancer screening.	http://www. americangeriatrics.org/ products/positionpapers/ cer_carc_2000.shtml J Am Geriatr Soc 2001;49:655
	CTF	1994				

[a]Risk factors for cervical cancer: sexual activity, early onset of sexual intercourse, history of multiple sexual partners, history of multiple sexual partners who have had multiple sexual partners, male partners whose other sexual partners have had cervical cancer, history of STDs (especially HPV, HIV, HSV), immunosuppression, smoking, history of cervical dysplasia or endometrial, vaginal, or vulvar cancer, and no previous screening (may indicate more frequent screening interval). (Am Intern Med 2000;133:1021–1024)
[http://www.cancernet.nci.nih.gov/clinpdq/screening; Ann Intern Med 1990;113(3):214]
[c]Long-term use of oral contraceptives may increase risk of cervical cancer in women who are positive for cervical human papillomavirus DNA. (Lancet 2002;359:1085)
[d]If sexual history is unknown or considered unreliable, screening should begin at age 18 years.
[e]New tests to improve cancer detection include liquid-based/thin-layer preparations, computer-assisted screening methods, and human papillomavirus testing. (Am Fam Phys 2001;64:729). None of these tests is currently recommended for routine screening.
The USPSTF, ACS, ACOG, and ASCO recommend *against* routine Pap smear screening in women who have had a total hysterectomy for benign disease and no history of abnormal cell growth.

CANCER, COLORECTAL

Disease Screening	Organization	Date	Population	Recommendations	Comments	Source
Cancer, Colorectal	ACG ACP AGA ASGE	2003	Aged ≥ 50 years at average risk[a]	Screen with 1 of the following strategies: 1) FOBT annually[b] 2) Flexible sigmoidoscopy every 5 years 3) FOBT annually plus flexible sigmoidoscopy every 5 years 4) Colonoscopy every 10 years 5) Double-contrast barium enema every 5 years	A positive screening test should be followed by colonoscopy.[c] Approximately half of patients with proximal neoplasms had no distal lesions.	Gastroenterology 2003;124:544 NEJM 2000;343:162 NEJM 2000;343:169
	ACS	2003	Aged ≥ 50 years[a]	See ACG, ACP, AGA, and ASGE recommendations for average risk persons above.	Yearly FOBT and flexible sigmoidoscopy is preferred to either alone. Patients should be involved in a shared decision-making process for choosing the most appropriate screening test.	CA Cancer J Clin 2001;51:38 http://caonline.amca ncersoc.org/cgi/con tent/full/51/1/38

CANCER, COLORECTAL

Disease Screening	Organization	Date	Population	Recommendations	Comments	Source
Cancer, Colorectal (continued)	USPSTF	2002	Aged > 50 years[a] Aged 50–80 years	Colorectal cancer screening with FOBT, flexible sigmoidoscopy alone, FOBT + flexible sigmoidoscopy, or colonoscopy is strongly recommended. There is insufficient evidence to recommend newer screening techniques (eg, CT colography). Guaiac-based FOBT[d,e] every 1–2 years. There is insufficient evidence to determine optimal interval of flexible sigmoidoscopy.	USPSTF did not find direct evidence that screening colonoscopy is effective in reducing colorectal cancer mortality rates. Models indicate that screening persons > 50 years for colorectal cancer with annual FOBT, flexible sigmoidoscopy, or a single colonoscopy compares favorably with screening mammography in women aged > 50 years in the cost per year of life saved. [NEJM 1995;332(13):861] Screening for colorectal cancer, even in the setting of imperfect compliance, significantly reduces colorectal cancer mortality at costs comparable to other cancer screening procedures. (JAMA 2000;284:1954–1961) Beginning in July 2001, Medicare will cover screening colonoscopy every 10 years for people who are NOT at high risk for colon cancer. (HCFA Press Release, 3/14/01; www.hcfa.gov) In a prospective study, one-time screening with FOBT and sigmoidoscopy fails to detect 24% of subjects with advanced colonic neoplasia. (NEJM 2001;345:555)	www.ahrq.gov/clinic/uspstf/uspscolo.htm Ann Intern Med 2002;137:129 http://cancernet.nci.nih.gov/

CANCER, COLORECTAL

Disease Screening	Organization	Date	Population	Recommendations	Comments	Source
Cancer, Colorectal (continued)	AAFP	2002	Aged ≥ 50 years	"Recommends, not strongly" Yearly FOBT,[c,f] flexible sigmoidoscopy, colonoscopy, or barium enema	If family H$_x$ of early colorectal cancer, begin screening at 40 years.	http://www.aafp.org/exam. xml
	ASCRS	1999	Aged ≥ 50 years, low or average risk[a]	Yearly DRE and 1 of the following: FOBT[d,e] and flexible sigmoidoscopy every 5 years OR Total colon exam (colonoscopy or double-contrast barium enema and proctosigmoidoscopy)		www.fascrs.org/
	ACG ACP AGA ASGE	2003	Persons at increased risk based on family history[f]	Group I: Screening colonoscopy at age 40 years, or 10 years younger than the earliest diagnosis in their family, and repeated every 5 years. Group II: Follow average risk recommendations, but begin at age 40 years. Group III: see Average Risk		

CANCER, COLORECTAL

[a]Risk factors indicating need for earlier/more frequent screening: personal history of colorectal cancer or adenomatous polyps, colorectal cancer or polyps in a first-degree relative < 60 years old or in a second-degree relative of any age, personal history of chronic inflammatory bowel disease, and family with hereditary colorectal cancer syndromes. [Ann Intern Med 1998;128(1):900, NEJM 1994;331(25):1669, NEJM 1995;332(13):861] If history of colorectal cancer in first-degree relative, age 55 years or younger, or 2 or more first-degree relatives of any ages, colonoscopy is recommended at age 40 or 10 years before the youngest case in the family, whichever is earlier. (http://www.fascrs.org)

[b]Use the guaiac-based test with dietary restriction, or an immunochemical test without dietary restriction. Two samples from each of 3 consecutive stools should be examined without rehydration. Rehydration increases the false-positive rate.

[c]Colonoscopy is the preferred test. If not available, double-contrast barium enema and flexible sigmoidoscopy should be performed.

[d]A positive result on an FOBT should be followed by colonoscopy. An alternative is flexible sigmoidoscopy and air-contrast BE.

[e]FOBT should be performed on 2 samples from 3 consecutive specimens obtained at home.

[f]Group I: First-degree relative with colon cancer or adenomatous polyps at age ≥ 60 years, or 2 first-degree relatives with colorectal cancer at any time. Group II: First-degree relative with colon cancer or adenomatous polyp at age ≥ 60 years, or 2 first-degree relatives with colorectal cancer. Group III: 1 second-degree or third-degree relative with colorectal cancer.

FOBT = fecal occult blood testing

Disease Screening	Organization	Date	Population	Recommendations	Comments	Source
Cancer, Endometrial	NCI	2002	All women	There is insufficient evidence that screening with endometrial sampling or transvaginal ultrasound decreases mortality.	Presence of endometrial cells in Pap test from postmenopausal women not taking exogenous hormones is abnormal and requires further evaluation. Endometrial thickness of < 4 mm on transvaginal ultrasound is associated with low risk of endometrial cancer. [Obstet Gynecol 1991;78(2):195]	http://cancernet.nci.nih.gov/
	ACS	2001	All women	Routine screening of women for endometrial cancer is not recommended.		CA Cancer J Clin 2001;51:54
	ACS	2001	All women at high risk for endometrial cancer.[a]	Annual screening at age 35 years with endometrial biopsy	Variable screening with ultrasound among women (aged 25–65 years; $n = 292$) at high risk for HNPCC mutation detected no cancers from ultrasound. Two endometrial causes occurred in the cohort that presented with symptoms. (Cancer 2002;94:1708) One should also consider that the RR of endometrial cancer associated with tamoxifen use in women with breast cancer is approximately 1.5 overall, and increases to RR = 6.9 for women taking tamoxifen at least 5 years. (Lancet 2000;356:881)	CA Cancer J Clin 2001;51:54

[a]High-risk women are those known to carry hereditary nonpolyposis colorectal cancer-associated genetic mutations, or at high risk to carry mutation, or who are from families with suspected autosomal dominant predisposition to colon cancer.

CANCER, GASTRIC						
Disease Screening	Organization	Date	Population	Recommendations	Comments	Source
Cancer, Gastric	NCI	2003	Adults in United States	There is insufficient evidence to establish that screening would result in a decrease in mortality from gastric cancer in the U.S. population.	Studies of screening in Japan (via barium x-ray) have demonstrated decreases in mortality in screened vs. unscreened patients. (Int J Cancer 1995;60:45)	http://cancernet.nci.nih.gov/

	CANCER, LIVER				

Disease Screening	Organization	Date	Population	Recommendations	Comments	Source
Cancer, Liver (Hepatocellular Carcinoma, HCC)	NCI	2003	Children and adults	There is insufficient evidence to establish that screening by alpha fetoprotein (AFP) and/or imaging techniques (eg, CT or ultrasound) would result in a decrease in mortality from HCC.	Chronic hepatitis B and C are the major risk factors for HCC. In the United States, chronic hepatitis B and C account for ~30%–40% of HCC. Other risk factors: alcoholic cirrhosis, hemochromatosis, alpha-1-antitrypsin deficiency, glycogen storage disease, porphyria cutanea tarda, tyrosinemia, Wilson's disease. 20%–50% of patients presenting with HCC have previously undiagnosed cirrhosis.	www.cancernet.nci.nih.gov
	British Society of Gastroenterology	2003	Adults	Surveillance with abdominal ultrasound and AFP every 6 months should be considered for high-risk groups[a]	Patients should be made aware of the implications of early diagnosis and lack of proven survival benefit. Patients with single small HCC (≤ 5 cm) or up to 3 lesions ≤ 3 cm should be referred for assessment for hepatic resection or transplantation.	Gut 2003;52(Suppl III):iii

[a] All persons with established cirrhosis with HBV, HCV, or hemachromatosis; males with cirrhosis due to alcohol or primary biliary cirrhosis.

CANCER, LUNG

Disease Screening	Organization	Date	Population	Recommendations	Comments	Source
Cancer, Lung	ACCP NCI AAFP ACS USPSTF CTF	2003 2003 2002 2002 1996 1994	Asymptomatic persons	Routine screening for lung cancer with CXR, sputum cytology, or low-dose CT (LDCT) is not recommended.	Counsel all patients against tobacco use. No significant benefit in terms of lung cancer mortality by screening with CXR and sputum cytology. (J Occup Med 1986;28:746) Annual low-dose chest CT in high-risk patients appears to increase detection of resectable cancer. Impact of screening on mortality has not been determined. (Lancet 1999;354:99–105) Although there is public and political pressure, based on low-dose CT prevalence-screening data, to change clinical practice and to offer mass lung-cancer screening, there should be no compromise or shortcuts in the rigorous scientific process required to determine whether this process is justified. (www.uicc.org, NEJM 2000;343:1627, JAMA 2000;284:1980) The NCI is conducting the National Lung Screening Test (NLST), an RCT comparing LDCT and CXR for detecting and reducing lung cancer mortality among persons at risk for lung cancer. (www.cancer.org)	http://cancernet.nci.nih.gov/ http://www.aafp.org/exam.xml www.cancer.org The Medical Letter 2001;43(1109):61–62 Chest 2003;123:835–885

CANCER, ORAL						

Disease Screening	Organization	Date	Population	Recommendations	Comments	Source
Cancer, Oral	NCI CTF USPSTF	2003 1999 1996	Asymptomatic persons	There is insufficient evidence to establish that screening would result in a decrease in mortality from oral cancer.		http://cancernet.nci.nih.gov/ J Can Dent Assoc 1999;65:617
	NIDR	1994	Asymptomatic persons	Screen during routine dental exam.		Detecting Oral Cancer: A Guide for Dentists. NIDR, 1994.
	CTF USPSTF	1999 1996	High-risk persons[a]	Consider annual oral exam.[b]		

[a]Risk factors: regular alcohol or tobacco use.
[b]Inquire about alcohol and tobacco use and counsel about risk.

				CANCER, OVARIAN		
Disease Screening	Organization	Date	Population	Recommendations	Comments	Source
Cancer, Ovarian	AAFP ASCO NCI ACPM USPSTF CTF	2003 2003 2003 1997 1996 1994	Asymptomatic women[a]	There is insufficient evidence to establish that screening for ovarian cancer with serum markers such as CA-125 levels, transvaginal ultrasound, or pelvic examinations would result in a decrease in mortality from ovarian cancer.	In asymptomatic women, pelvic exam has unknown sensitivity and specificity; abdominal ultrasound has specificity 97.7%, sensitivity 100%, positive predictive value 2.6%; transvaginal ultrasound has specificity 98.1%, sensitivity 100%, positive predictive value 22%; CA-125 has sensitivity 50% for stages I and II and 90% for stages III and IV, and specificity 97.6%, when followed by abdominal ultrasound. [Ann Intern Med 1993;118(11):838; http://www.acpm.org/ovary.htm]	www.aafp.org/exam.xml www.asco.org http://www.cancernet.nci.nih.gov/ www.acpm.org/ovary.htm
	ACOG ASCO ACS	2003 2003 2002	Asymptomatic women[a]	Recommend physical examination every 3 years in women aged 20–39 years, and annually in women aged ≥ 40 years.		www.acog.org www.asco.org CA Cancer J Clin 2002;52:8
	NIH	1994	Asymptomatic women[a]	Comprehensive family history and annual rectovaginal pelvic exam		NIH Consensus Statement 1994;12(3):1

CANCER, OVARIAN

[a]Risk factors: aged > 60 years; low parity; personal history of endometrial, colon, or breast cancer; family history of ovarian cancer; and hereditary ovarian cancer syndrome. Lifetime risk of ovarian cancer in a woman with no affected relatives is 1 in 70. If 1 first-degree relative has ovarian cancer, lifetime risk is 5%. If 2 or more first-degree relatives have ovarian cancer, lifetime risk is 7%. Women with 2 or more family members affected by ovarian cancer have a 3% chance of having a hereditary ovarian cancer syndrome. These women have a 40% lifetime risk of ovarian cancer. There are no data demonstrating that screening high-risk women reduces their mortality from ovarian cancer. A low annual incidence (13.8/100,000) means that many people must be screened to find only a few cases of disease. [NIH Consensus Statement 1994;12(3):1, Ann Intern Med 1993;118(11):838]

Several large-scale studies designed to establish the effectiveness of general population screening for ovarian cancer have begun. Each uses transvaginal ultrasonography or a multimodal strategy in which elevated serum levels of CA-125 tumor marker prompt secondary testing with transvaginal ultrasonography. (Ann Intern Med 2000;133:1021–1024)

CANCER, PANCREATIC					

Disease Screening	Organization	Date	Population	Recommendations	Comments	Source
Cancer, Pancreatic	AAFP USPSTF CTF	2002 1996 1994	Asymptomatic persons	Routine screening using abdominal palpation, ultrasonography, or serologic markers is not recommended.	Cigarette smoking has consistently been associated with increased risk of pancreatic cancer.	www.aafp.org/exam.xml

CANCER, PROSTATE					
Disease Screening	Organization	Date	Population	Recommendations	Comments	Source
Cancer, Prostate	NCI	2003	Asymptomatic men	Insufficient evidence to establish whether a decrease in mortality from prostate cancer occurs with screening by DRE or serum PSA.	Although some observational studies have witnessed a fall in prostate cancer mortality among screened individuals, these observations have not been consistent in all populations or within a given population.	http://cancernet.nci. nih.gov/
	USPSTF	2002	Asymptomatic men	Evidence insufficient to recommend for or against routine screening using PSA or DRE.	There is good evidence that PSA can detect early-stage prostate cancer, but mixed and inconclusive evidence that early detection improves health outcomes.	
	ACS AUA	2002 2001	Men aged ≥ 50 years[a]	Offer annual PSA and DRE if > 10-year life expectancy.[b]	DRE has sensitivity 50%, specificity 94%; PSA has sensitivity 67%, specificity 84%; TRUS has sensitivity 81%, specificity 84%. [JAMA 1994;272(10):773]	www.cancer.org Oncology 2000; 14:267–286 http://amanet.org
	AAFP	2002	Men aged 50–65 years	Recommends, but not strongly. Counsel regarding the known risks and uncertain benefits of screening for prostate cancer.		http://www.aafp. org/exam.xml

CANCER, PROSTATE					
Disease Screening	Organization	Date	Population	Recommendations	Comments	Source
Cancer, Prostate (continued)	ACPM ACP	1998 1997	Men aged > 50 years[a]	Describe potential benefits and known harms of screening with PSA and DRE, diagnosis, and treatment; listen to the patient's concerns; and individualize the decision to screen.	Data are not yet available to quantify the risks and benefits of screening for prostate cancer or to prove that treating clinically localized cancer reduces disease-specific mortality rates. [Ann Intern Med 1997;126(6):468]	www.acpm.org/prostate.htm Ann Intern Med 1997;126(6):480

[a]Men in high-risk groups (2 or more affected first-degree relatives, blacks) should begin screening at age 40. If PSA < 1.0 ng/mL, no additional testing is needed until age 45. If PSA 1.0–2.5 ng/mL, annual testing is recommended. If PSA ≥ 2.5 ng/mL, consider further evaluation with biopsy. More data on the precise age to start prostate cancer screening are needed for men at high risk. No direct or indirect evidence quantifies the yield and predictive value of early detection efforts in higher-risk men. [http://www.cancer.org/, http://auanet.org/pub_pat/policies/uroservices.html, Ann Intern Med 1997;126(6):480]

[b]Some elevations in PSA may be due to benign conditions of the prostate. The DRE should be performed by health care workers skilled in recognizing subtle prostate abnormalities, including those of symmetry and consistency, as well as the more classic findings of marked induration or nodules. DRE is less effective in detecting prostate carcinoma than is PSA. (http://www.cancer.org/, http://auanet.org/)

Disease Screening	Organization	Date	Population	Recommendations	Comments	Source
Cancer, Skin	NCI AAFP USPSTF CTF	2003 2002 1996 1994	Asymptomatic persons	Insufficient evidence to recommend for or against routine screening using total-body skin exam[a] OR Counseling patients to perform periodic skin self-exam.[b]		http://cancernet.nci.nih.gov/ www.aafp.org/exam.xml
	ACPM	1998	Asymptomatic persons	Periodic total cutaneous examinations, targeting populations at high risk for malignant melanoma.[b] Insufficient evidence to characterize periodicity of skin examinations more precisely.		http://www.acpm.org/ skincanc.htm
	AAD	1992	Asymptomatic persons	Annual screening using total-body skin exam.		J Am Acad Dermatol 1992;26:629
	ACS	2003	Aged 20–39 years	Screening with physician skin exam every 3 years		www.cancer.org
	ACS	2003	Aged ≥ 40 years	Annual screening with physician skin exam		www.cancer.org

[a]Clinicians should remain alert for skin lesions with malignant features when examining patients for other reasons, particularly patients with established risk factors. Risk factors for skin cancer include: evidence of melanocytic precursors, large numbers of common moles, immunosuppression, family or personal history of skin cancer, substantial cumulative lifetime sun exposure, intermittent intense sun exposure or severe sunburns in childhood, freckles, poor tanning ability, and light skin, hair, and eye color. Appropriate biopsy specimens should be taken of suspicious lesions. Persons with melanocytic precursor or marker lesions are at substantially increased risk for malignant melanoma and should be referred to skin cancer specialists for evaluation and surveillance. (USPSTF)

[b]Consider educating patients with established risk factors for skin cancer (see above) concerning signs and symptoms suggesting skin cancer and the possible benefits of periodic self-exam. (USPSTF)

Disease Screening	Organization	Date	Population	Recommendations	Comments	Source
Cancer, Testicular	NCI USPSTF CTF	2003 1996 1994	Asymptomatic men[a]	Insufficient evidence to recommend for or against routine screening by physician exam, patient self-exam, or tumor markers (alpha fetoprotein, human chorionic gonadotropin). Insufficient evidence to establish that screening would result in a decrease in mortality from testicular cancer.		http://cancernet.nci.nih.gov/

[a]Patients with history of cryptorchidism, orchiopexy, or testicular atrophy should be informed of their increased risk for developing testicular cancer and counseled about screening. Such patients may then elect to be screened or to perform testicular self-exam. Adolescent and young adult males should be advised to seek prompt medical attention if they notice a scrotal abnormality. (USPSTF)

| **CANCER, THYROID** | | | | | |

Disease Screening	Organization	Date	Population	Recommendations	Comments	Source
Cancer, Thyroid	AAFP USPSTF CTF	2002 1996 1994	Asymptomatic persons	Screening asymptomatic adults or children using either neck palpation or ultrasonography is not recommended.[a]	Neck palpation for nodules in asymptomatic individuals has sensitivity 15%–38%; specificity 93%–100%. Only a small proportion of nodular thyroid glands are neoplastic, resulting in a high false-positive rate. (USPSTF)	www.aafp.org/exam.xml

[a]Includes asymptomatic persons with a history of external upper-body irradiation in infancy or childhood.

	CAROTID ARTERY STENOSIS					
Disease Screening	Organization	Date	Population	Recommendations	Comments	Source
Carotid Artery Stenosis (asymptomatic)	AHA	1998	Aged 40–79 years	Screen asymptomatic patients (? interval) with < 5% surgical risk and > 5-year life expectancy.[a]	In the Asymptomatic Carotid Atherosclerosis Study (ACAS), the actuarial 5-year risk of ipsilateral stroke, operative stroke, and death was ≅ 5% with CEA vs. 11% in the control group. Combined surgical morbidity and mortality was 2.3%. (JAMA 1995;273:1421) In ACAS, the benefit of surgery was greater for men than women (reduction in risk 66% vs. 17%).	http://circ.ahajournals.org/cgi/content/full/97/5/501
	CNS	1997	Aged 40–79 years	Insufficient evidence to screen asymptomatic individuals because CEA recommendation is "uncertain" for > 60% stenosis.[b]		Can Med Assoc J 1997;157:653
	USPSTF	1996	Aged > 60 years	Selective screening.[c]	The cumulative cost-effectiveness of targeted screening and surgery for high-grade carotid artery stenosis is ~$43,000 per QALY. (MJM 1999;5:35–41)	

CAROTID ARTERY STENOSIS					
Disease Screening	**Organization**	**Date**	**Population**	**Recommendations**	**Source**
Carotid Artery Stenosis (asymptomatic) (continued)	SVU	2000		Insufficient evidence to recommend screening asymptomatic individuals. Selective screening[d]	www.svunet.org

Comments: The prevalence of internal carotid artery stenosis (ICAS) of ≥ 70% is low in persons with only atherosclerosis risk factors (1.8%–2.3%), intermediate in those with angina or MI (3.1%), and highest in those with PAD (12.5%) or AAA (8.8%). Advanced age (> 54 years) and lower diastolic BP (<83 mm HG) increased prevalence of ICAS. (*J Vasc Surg* 2003;37: 1226–1233)

	CTF	1994		Insufficient evidence to screen	

[a]If surgical risk is < 3% and life expectancy is > 5 years, ipsilateral CEA is acceptable for > 60% stenosis; if surgical risk is 35%, ipsilateral CEA is acceptable (but not proved) for > 75% bilateral stenoses.

[b]Recommend stenosis be documented with angiography using the method of the North American Symptomatic Carotid Endarterectomy Trial.

[c]Selective screening may be appropriate in the presence of other stroke risk factors, no contraindications to major surgery, and access to surgeons and centers with < 3% perioperative morbidity and mortality.

[d]Screen patients with audible carotid bruit, multiple risk factors for CAS, or those who are preparing for operation in another vascular bed using duplex scan. Recommend CEA for patients with > 75% stenosis with life expectancy > 5 years and surgical risk < 3%. Other candidates for CEA include those with CT scan evidence of silent embolization, mixed plaque consistency, or evidence that the lesion has progressed over 6 months.

CHILD ABUSE & NEGLECT					
Disease Screening	Organization	Date	Population	Recommendations	Comments	Source
Child Abuse & Neglect	GAPS	1997	Children and adolescents	All teens should be asked annually about a history of emotional, physical, and sexual abuse.	By law, child abuse must be reported to appropriate authorities in all 50 states.	Arch Pediatr Adolesc Med 1997;151:123

CHLAMYDIAL INFECTION

Disease Screening	Organization	Date	Population	Recommendations	Comments	Source
Chlamydial Infection	ACPM	2003	Sexually active women	Annually screen high-risk women[a]	When economically feasible, amplified tests are preferred.	Am J Prev Med 2003;24:287
	AAFP	2002	Women ≤ 25 who are sexually active	Strongly recommends screening		
	USPSTF	2001	Women aged ≤ 25 years who are sexually active or pregnant	Routinely screen for chlamydial infection; the optimal interval for screening is uncertain[b]	Antigen detection tests and nonamplified nucleic acid hybridization, as well as newer amplified DNA assays, may provide improved sensitivity, lower expense, availability, and/or timeliness of results over culture. Noninvasive methods such as urine specimens and vaginal swabs appear reliable. Early detection and treatment of women at risk for chlamydial infection (prevalence 7%) reduced the incidence of pelvic inflammatory disease from 28 per 1,000 woman-years to 13 per 1,000 woman-years. Ecologic studies also show a decrease in ectopic pregnancy with the advent of community-based chlamydial screening programs.	Am J Prev Med 2001;20(3S):90
	ACPM	2003	Pregnant women	Screen during their first trimester or first prenatal visit		Am J Prev Med 2003;24:287

[a] Aged ≤ 25 years, new male sex partner or 2 or more partners during preceding year, inconsistent use of barrier methods, history of prior STD, African-American race, cervical ectopy.
[b] For women with a previous negative screening test, the interval for rescreening should take into account changes in sexual partners. If there is evidence that a woman is at low risk for infection (eg, in a mutually monogamous relationship with a previous history of negative screening tests for chlamydial infection), it may not be necessary to screen frequently. Rescreening at 6 to 12 months may be appropriate for previously infected women because of high rates of reinfection.

	CHOLESTEROL & LIPID DISORDERS, CHILDREN					
Disease Screening	Organization	Date	Population	Recommendations	Comments	Source
Cholesterol & Lipid Disorders, Children	AAP	1998	Aged > 2 years	Selective screening[a] every 5 years if normal[b] Fasting lipids if strong family history Random total cholesterol if a parent has total cholesterol ≥ 240 mg/dL. Clinician discretion (random total cholesterol) if unknown family history or presence of risk factors	Recommend pharmacologic treatment (eg, cholestyramine or colestipol) if: (1) age > 10 years, on dietary therapy, and LDL ≥ 190 mg/dL without other risk factors; or (2) LDL ≥ 160 mg/dL and strong family history or 2 or more risk factors are present.[a] See management algorithms.	Pediatrics 1998;101: 141–147
	USPSTF	1996	Children and adolescents	Insufficient evidence to recommend for or against screening		
	GAPS	1994	Aged > 2 years	See AAP/NCEP recommendations; measure cholesterol only once if normal		

	CHOLESTEROL & LIPID DISORDERS, ADULTS				
Disease Screening	Organization	Date	Population	Recommendations	Comments	Source
Cholesterol & Lipid Disorders, Adults	NCEP III	2002	Men and women aged > 20 years	Check fasting lipoprotein panel (if testing opportunity is non-fasting, use TC and HDL) every 5 years if in desirable range; otherwise see management algorithm. [b]	NCEP III modifies recommendations (vs. NCEP II) to promote more aggressive primary prevention (ie, intensive lipid lowering) in persons with multiple risk factors for CHD.	Circulation 2002;106:3143
	USPSTF AAFP	2001	Men aged 20–35 years Women aged 20–45 years	Selective screening of individuals with major CHD risk factors [hypertension, smoking, diabetes, family history of CHD before age 50 (♂ relatives) or age 60 (♀ relatives), family history suggestive of familial hyperlipidemia]	Optimal interval for screening is uncertain.	
	ACP	1996	Men aged < 35 years Women aged < 45 years	Screening not recommended unless history or physical exam suggests familial lipoprotein disorder, or at least 2 other CHD risk factors are present.		Ann Intern Med 1996;124:515

CHOLESTEROL & LIPID DISORDERS, ADULTS

Disease Screening	Organization	Date	Population	Recommendations	Comments	Source
Cholesterol & Lipid Disorders, Adults (continued)	AAFP USPSTF	2002 2001	Men aged ≥ 35 years Women aged ≥ 45 years	"Strongly recommended" Random total cholesterol and HDL cholesterol or fasting lipid profile, periodicity based on risk factors	Base treatment decisions on at least 2 cholesterol levels. Age to stop screening is not established.	Am J Prev Med 2001;20(35):73–76 http://www.aafp.org/exam.xml
	ACP	1996	Men aged 35–65 years Women aged 45–65 years	"Appropriate but not mandatory"; random total cholesterol every 5 years if normal	Recommendations were published before 2 large primary prevention trials with HMG-CoA reductase inhibitors demonstrated efficacy and safety. (Lancet 1994;344:1383, NEJM 1995;333:1301) Base treatment decisions on at least 2 cholesterol levels.	
	ACP	1996	Men and women aged 66–75 years	Insufficient evidence to recommend for or against screening		
	ACP	1996	Men and women aged > 75 years	Screening not recommended		

[a] AAP recommends annual screening if strong family history (parents or grandparents) of cardiovascular events at or before age 55 years (MI, positive coronary angiogram, stroke, peripheral vascular disease, or sudden cardiac death) or presence of "several" risk factors (cigarette smoking, hypertension, obesity, diabetes, lack of physical activity).
[b] Classify TC < 200 mg/dL as desirable, 200–239 mg/dL as borderline, or ≥ 240 mg/dL as high. Classify HDL < 40 as low, and ≥ 60 as high. Classify LDL < 100 as optimal, 100–129 as near or above optimal, 130–159 as borderline high, 160–189 as high, and ≥ 190 as very high. If TC < 200 mg/dL and HDL ≥ 40 mg/dL, then repeat in 5 years; if TC ≥ 200 mg/dL or HDL < 40 mg/dL, then check fasting lipids and risk stratify based on LDL (see management algorithm).

DEMENTIA						

Disease Screening	Organization	Date	Population	Recommendations	Comments	Source
Dementia	AHCPR	1996	Elderly	Perform selective screening[a] using a standardized instrument to assess cognitive function (see Mini Mental State Examination in Appendix I).[b]	Screening instruments are useful for detecting multiple cognitive deficits and determining a baseline for future assessments. Reversible causes of dementia include vitamin B_{12} deficiency, neurosyphilis, and hypothyroidism. The additional benefit of identifying early dementia is to prepare family for future patient needs.	J Am Geriatr Soc 1988;37:562 Activities of daily living: J Am Geriatr Soc 1985;33:698 Mini Mental Status Exam: J Psychiatr Res 1975;12:189, see p. 155
	USPSTF CTF	2003 2001	Elderly, asymptomatic	Insufficient evidence to recommend for or against routine screening for dementia in older adults	Remain alert for signs of declining cognitive function.[a] Be aware of other causes of mental status changes, such as depression, delirium, medication effects, and coexisting illnesses.	Ann Intern Med 2003;138:925–926 Ann Intern Med 2003;138:927–937
	AGS AAN	2003 2001	Elderly, Mild Cognitive Impairment (MCI)[c]	Persons with MCI should be evaluated regularly for progression to dementia.		www.aan.org www.americangeriatrics.org

[a]Triggers that should initiate an assessment for dementia include difficulties in (1) learning and retaining new information, (2) handling complex tasks (eg, balancing a checkbook or cooking a meal), (3) reasoning ability (eg, a new disregard for social norms), (4) spatial ability and orientation (eg, difficulty driving, or getting lost), (5) language (eg, difficulties in word-finding, and (6) behavior (eg, appearing more passive or more irritable than usual).
[b]DSM-IV diagnosis of dementia requires: (1) evidence of decline in functional abilities and (2) evidence of multiple cognitive deficiencies.
[c]MCI is a classification of persons with memory impairment who are not demented (normal cognitive function, intact activities of daily living). 6%–25% of MCI patients progress to dementia each year.

	DEPRESSION					
Disease Screening	**Organization**	**Date**	**Population**	**Recommendations**	**Comments**	**Source**
Depression	USPSTF	2002	Children and adolescents	Insufficient evidence to recommend for or against routine screening		
	Bright Futures GAPS	2002 1994	Adolescents	Annual screening for behaviors or emotions that might indicate depression or risk of suicide	Clues to depression include poor school performance, alcohol or drug use, and deteriorating parental or peer relationships. Clues to suicide risk include family dysfunction, physical and sexual abuse, substance abuse, history of recurrent or severe depression, and prior suicide attempt or plans.[a]	
	USPSTF	2002	Adults	Screen adults in practices that have systems in place to assure accurate diagnosis, effective treatment, and follow-up.	Asking 2 simple questions may be as effective as longer instruments (see Appendix I). (J Gen Intern Med 1997;12:439) • Over the past 2 weeks, have you felt down, depressed, or hopeless? • Over the past 2 weeks, have you felt little interest or pleasure in doing things? Optimal screening interval is unknown.	http://www.ahrq.gov/ clinic/cpgsix.htm

Disease Screening	Organization	Date	Population	Recommendations	Comments	Source
DEPRESSION						
Depression (continued)	AHCPR	1993	Adults	Selective screening when risk factors are present.[b,c]	See screening instruments [Geriatric Depression Scale, Beck Depression Inventory (Short Form), PRIME-MD] in Appendix I.	Clinical Practice Guideline No. 5: Depression in Primary Care. Agency for Healthcare Policy and Research; 1993. AHCPR Publication 93-0550 Arch Gen Psychiatry 1998;55:1121

[a]Suicide risk increases as the number of conditions increases. Parents of adolescents at risk for suicide should reduce access to firearms, weapons, or potentially lethal drugs in the home.

[b]Risk factors include prior episodes of depression, family history (first-degree relative) of depressive disorder, prior suicide attempts, age < 40 years, female gender, postpartum period, medical comorbidity, lack of social support, stressful life events, and current alcohol or substance abuse.

[c]Suspicion or documentation of depression by history should lead to a mental status exam that includes documentation of suicidal ideation; level of orientation, alertness, cooperation, and communication; level of motor activity; and presence or absence of psychotic features.

DIABETES MELLITUS, GESTATIONAL					
Disease Screening	Organization	Date	Population	Recommendations	Comments	Source
Diabetes Mellitus, Gestational (GDM)	USPSTF	2003	Pregnant women	Evidence is insufficient to recommend for or against screening.	This is insufficient evidence that screening GDM substantially reduces important adverse health outcomes for mothers or their infants.	
	ACOG	2001	Pregnant women	Screen all pregnant women for GDM by patient history, clinical risk factors, and laboratory test.[a]		www.acog.org
	ADA	1998	Pregnant women	Risk assessment for GDM at first prenatal visit. If clinical characteristics consistent with a high risk of GDM[b] do glucose testing as soon as possible. If no GDM at initial testing, retest between 24–28 weeks' gestation. Average-risk women: test at 24–28 weeks' gestation. Low-risk women[c]: no glucose testing.	Positive 1-hour OGTT: serum glucose > 140 mg/dL after 50 g oral glucose Confirmation test: 3-hour OGTT	Diabetes Care 2002;25:94–96 Diabetes Care 2003;26(Suppl): 103

				DIABETES MELLITUS, TYPE 2		
Disease Screening	Organization	Date	Population	Recommendations	Comments	Source
Diabetes Mellitus, Type 2	ADA	2003	Adults	Screen with fasting glucose at 3-year intervals beginning at age 45; consider testing earlier or more frequently in overweight patients if diabetes risk factors present.[c]	Screening appears to be more cost-effective for younger people (aged 25–45 years) and blacks. Impaired fasting glucose: ≥ 110 and < 126 mg/dL. Impaired glucose tolerance: 2 hour PG ≥ 140 and < 200 g/dL. Diabetes defined as fasting glucose ≥ 126 mg/dL on 2 separate occasions, or symptoms of diabetes with random glucose ≥ 200 mg/dL.	Diabetes Care 2003;26 (Suppl):S23
	USPSTF	2003	Adults	Evidence is insufficient to recommend for or against screening asymptomatic adults for type 2 diabetes, impaired glucose tolerance, or impaired fasting glucose.	It has not been demonstrated that beginning diabetes control early as a result of screening provides an incremental benefit compared with initiating treatment after clinical diagnosis.	
	USPSTF	2003	Hypertensive or hyperlipidemic adults	Recommends screening (test and frequency not known).	In hypertensives, there is strong evidence that more aggressive blood pressure control is beneficial when diabetes is present. In hyperlipidemia, NCEP III recommends different treatment thresholds and targets when diabetes is present.	

[a]Low risk for GDM (may *not* need lab screening): < 25 years old; not Hispanic, African, Native American, South or East Asian, Pacific Islands ancestry; BMI ≤ 25; no history of abnormal glucose tolerance; no previous history of adverse pregnancy outcomes usually associated with GDM; no known diabetes in first-degree relative.
[b]High risk is defined as (1) obesity (BMI > 27 kg/m^2) (see BMI Conversion Table in Appendix IV), (2) strong family history of diabetes, (3) personal history of GDM, or (4) glycosuria.
[c]Risk factors (in addition to age ≥ 45 years) include (1) family history of diabetes in parents or siblings, (2) membership in one of the following ethnic groups: African-American, Hispanic-American, Native American, Asian American, or Pacific Islander, (3) history of impaired fasting glucose, impaired glucose tolerance, gestational diabetes, or mother with infant birthweight > 9 lb, (4) comorbid conditions, including hypertension (> 140/90 mm Hg) or dyslipidemia (HDL < 35 mg/dL or TGs > 250 mg/dL), (5) overweight (BMI ≥ 25 kg/m^2), (6) polycystic ovary syndrome, and (7) history of vascular disease.

DOMESTIC VIOLENCE & ABUSE						
Disease Screening	**Organization**	**Date**	**Population**	**Recommendations**	**Comments**	**Source**
Domestic (Intimate Partner) Violence & Abuse	ACOG	1996	Women	Recommend routine, direct questions about domestic violence.[a]	Controversy exists regarding the overall benefit of mandatory reporting of domestic violence. (JAMA 1995; 273:1781) Barriers to screening include lack of provider education and time. Interventions that incorporated strategies in addition to provider education (eg, providing specific screening questions) were associated with significant increases in identification rates. (Am J Prev Med 2000;19:230)	www.acog.org
	ACOG	1996	Elderly		Some states have mandatory reporting of elder abuse and neglect.	

[a]Recommended questions: (1) Within the past year—or since you have been pregnant—have you been hit, slapped, kicked, or otherwise physically hurt by someone?; (2) Are you in a relationship with a person who threatens or physically hurts you?; (3) Has anyone forced you to have sexual activities that made you feel uncomfortable?

FALLS IN THE ELDERLY						
Disease Screening	Organization	Date	Population	Recommendations	Comments	Source
Falls in the Elderly	AGS British Geriatrics Society AAOS	2001	All older persons	Ask at least yearly about falls.[a]	See also page 76 for fall prevention and Appendix II.	JAGS 2001;49:664–672
	USPSTF	1996	All persons aged ≥ 75 years and those aged 70–74 years with a known risk factor[b]	Counsel about specific measures to prevent falls.		

[a]All who report a single fall should be observed as they stand up from a chair without using their arms, walk several paces, and return (see Appendix II, page 161). Those demonstrating no difficulty or unsteadiness need no further assessment. Those who have difficulty or demonstrate unsteadiness, have ≥ 1 fall, or present for medical attention after a fall should have a fall evaluation, see Fall Prevention, page 76).

[b]Risk factors: Intrinsic: lower extremity weakness, poor grip strength, balance disorders, functional and cognitive impairment, visual deficits. Extrinsic: polypharmacy (≥ 4 prescription medications), environment (poor lighting, loose carpets, lack of bathroom safety equipment).

Disease Screening	Organization	Date	Population	Recommendations	Comments	Source
Hearing Impairment	Bright Futures Joint Committee on Infant Hearing[a] AAP	2002 2000 2000	Infants	The hearing of all infants should be screened using objective, physiologic measures to identify those with congenital or neonatal onset hearing loss. Audiologic evaluations should be in progress before 3 months of age. Infants with confirmed hearing loss should receive intervention before 6 months of age.	The efficacy of universal newborn hearing screening to improve long-term language outcomes remains uncertain. (JAMA 2001;286:2000–2010)	Pediatrics 2000;106(4):798–817 www.aap.org
	AAFP USPSTF CTF	2002 2001 1994	Normal-risk infants and children	Insufficient evidence to recommend for or against routine screening of neonates. Routine screening beyond age 3 years is not recommended.		www.aafp.org/exam.xml www.ahrq.gov/clinic/cpgsix.htm Am Fam Physician 2001;64(12):1995–1999
	AAP Bright Futures USPSTF Joint Committee on Infant Hearing[a]	2003 2002 2000 1996	High-risk infants and children[b,c]	Infants should be screened no later than 3 months of age. Screen infants and children < 2 years of age with increased risk. Screen every 6 months until 3 years of age and at appropriate intervals thereafter if there is risk for delayed-onset hearing loss.		Pediatrics 2000;106(4):798–817 www.aap.org Pediatrics 2002;111:436–440

HEARING IMPAIRMENT

HEARING IMPAIRMENT

Disease Screening	Organization	Date	Population	Recommendations	Comments	Source
Hearing Impairment (continued)	AAP ASHA	2003 1994	High-risk children[c]	Children with frequent recurrent otitis media or middle-ear effusion, or both, should have audiology screening and monitoring of communication-skills development.		www.aap.org www.asha.org Pediatrics 2003;11:436–440
	Bright Futures	2002	Adolescents	Assess annually: screen with objective method at age 12 or more frequently if indicated		
	AAFP AGS USPSTF CTF	2002 1997 1997 1994	Adults	Question older adults periodically about hearing impairment, counsel about availability of hearing-aid devices, and make referrals for abnormalities when appropriate.	Older adults can be screened for hearing loss using simple methods. (JAMA 2003;289:1976–1985) (See also Appendix II: Functional Assessment Screening in the Elderly)	http://www.aafp.org/exam.xml www.ctfphc.org J Am Geriatr Soc 1997;45:344

[a]Joint Committee on Infant Hearing member organizations: American Academy of Audiology; American Academy of Otolaryngology–Head and Neck Surgery; American Academy of Pediatrics; American Speech-Language-Hearing Association; Council on Education of the Deaf; Directors of Speech and Hearing Programs in State Health and Welfare Agencies.

[b]Increased neonatal risk: family history of hereditary sensorineural hearing loss, intrauterine infection, craniofacial anomalies, birthweight < 1,500 g, hyperbilirubinemia requiring exchange transfusions, ototoxic medications, bacterial meningitis, Apgar scores 0–4 and 0–6, mechanical ventilation lasting > 5 days, and stigmata associated with a syndrome known to include hearing loss.

[c]Increased childhood risk: patient/caregiver concern regarding hearing, speech, language, or developmental delay; bacterial meningitis; head trauma associated with loss of consciousness or skull fracture; stigmata associated with a syndrome known to include hearing loss; ototoxic medications; recurrent or persistent otitis media with effusion; disorders affecting eustachian tube function; neurofibromatosis type 2; and neurodegenerative disorders. Delayed-onset hearing loss: as above for increased childhood risk plus family history of hereditary childhood hearing loss and intrauterine infection.

HEPATITIS B VIRUS

Disease Screening	Organization	Date	Population	Recommendations	Comments	Source
Hepatitis B Virus Infection, Chronic	CDC USPSTF ACP	2003 1996 1994	Pregnant women	Screen all women with HBsAg[a] at first prenatal visit. Repeat in third trimester if woman is initially HBsAg negative and engages in high-risk behavior.[b]	Screening all pregnant women in the United States each year is estimated to detect 22,000 HBsAg-positive mothers, and treatment of their newborns would prevent chronic HBV infection in 6,000 neonates per year. (Pediatr Infect Dis J 1992;11:866)	MMWR 1991;40(RR-13):1 Int J Gynaecol Obstet 1993;40:172
	USPSTF ACP	1996 1994	General population	Routine screening is not recommended.		
	USPSTF ACP	1997 1996	High-risk persons[b]	Insufficient evidence to recommend for or against screening to determine eligibility for vaccination, but recommendations for screening may be made based on cost-effectiveness analyses.		

[a]Immunoassays for HBsAg have sensitivity and specificity > 98%. (MMWR 1993;42:707)
[b]High risk includes injection drug users, sexual contact with HBV-infected persons or with persons at high risk for HBV infection, multiple sexual partners, and male homosexual activity.

HEPATITIS C VIRUS

Disease Screening	Organization	Date	Population	Recommendations	Comments	Source
Hepatitis C Virus Infection, Chronic	CDC AAP	2003 1998	Persons at increased risk[a]	Perform routine counseling, testing, and appropriate follow-up.[b] See algorithm on page 49.	15%–25% of persons with acute hepatitis C resolve their infection; of the remaining, 10%–20% develop cirrhosis and 1%–5% develop hepatocellular carcinoma. Abstinence from alcohol is imperative in patients with chronic hepatitis C.	MMWR 2003;52(RR-1) Pediatrics 1998;101(3):481

[a]Increased risk includes injection drug use, receipt of clotting factor concentrates before 1987, chronic hemodialysis, persistently abnormal alanine aminotransferase levels, receipt of blood from a donor who later tested positive for HCV, receipt of blood transfusion or blood components before July 1992, receipt of organ transplant before July 1992, health care workers after needle sticks or mucosal exposures to HCV-positive blood, and children born to HCV-positive women.
[b]2 types of tests are available for laboratory diagnosis of HCV infection: (1) detection of antibody to HCV antigens, and (2) detection and quantification of HCV nucleic acid. See algorithm on page 49.

HCV INFECTION TESTING ALGORITHM FOR ASYMPTOMATIC PERSONS

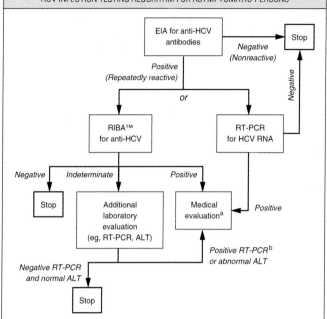

ALT = alanine aminotransferase; anti-HCV = antibody to HCV; EIA = enzyme immunoassay; RIBA™ = recombinant immunoblot assay; RT-PCR = reverse transcriptase polymerase chain reaction

[a]For possible anti-inflammatory and antiviral treatments.

[b]Treatment with combination peg-interferon alfa-2b plus ribavirin leads to sustained virologic response in about 50% of patients with detectable HCV RNA *and* elevated ALT. (Lancet 2001;358:958) Some liver disease specialists recommend liver biopsy and appropriate treatment in all patients with detectable HCV RNA, regardless of ALT levels. (Hepatology 2001;33:196)

Source: Adapted from MMWR 1998;47(RR-19):1.

					HUMAN IMMUNODEFICIENCY VIRUS	
Disease Screening	Organization	Date	Population	Recommendations	Comments	Source
Human Immunodeficiency Virus	CDC	2001	People at increased risk[a]	Routine and targeted counseling, testing, and referral (CTR) for HIV disease should be based on type of clinical setting, HIV prevalence in setting, and behavioral and clinical risk of individual clients in the setting. CTR should protect client confidentiality and be voluntary with informed consent. Provide patients with option for anonymous testing, written materials about HIV testing.	Confidential and anonymous voluntary testing is encouraged. Informed consent is needed. HIV prevention counseling focuses on client's own risk. CTR is targeted efficiently through risk screening.	MMWR 50(RR19):1
	AAFP Bright Futures USPSTF ACP GAPS CTF AAP AMA ACOG	2002 2002 1996 1994 1994 1994 1993 1993 1992	People at increased risk[a]	Counseling and testing for HIV should be offered.	Initial screening test: EIA is considered reactive only when a positive result is confirmed in a second test of the original sample. Seroconversion is 95% within 6 months of infection. Specificity is > 99.5%. False-positives with EIA: nonspecific reactions in persons with immunologic disturbances (eg, systemic lupus erythematosus or rheumatoid arthritis), multiple transfusions, recent influenza, or rabies vaccination. Confirmatory testing is necessary using Western blot or indirect immuno-fluorescence assay. Home tests available.[b]	Pediatrics 1993;92:626 MMWR 1987;36:509 Ann Intern Med 1994;120:310 Pediatrics 1995;95(2):303 www.aafp.org/exam.xml AMA: HIV Blood Test Counseling. Physician Guidelines. 2nd ed. AMA, 1993.

HUMAN IMMUNODEFICIENCY VIRUS

Disease Screening	Organization	Date	Population	Recommendations	Comments	Source
Human Immunodeficiency Virus (continued)	AAFP CDC ACOG	2001 2001 2000	Pregnant women	Universal testing with patient notification of all pregnant women (ie, testing is routinely performed unless patient actively refuses). Consent to testing should be in writing. Retest high-risk women at 36 weeks' gestation.	Pretest counseling modified to alleviate this burdensome barrier to testing as recommended by the Institute of Medicine Report. HIV testing as a routine part of antenatal care increased screening rates from 75% to 88%. (Obstet Gynecol 2001;98:1104)	MMWR 2001;50(RR19):59 Pediatrics 1995;95:303 NEJM 1994;331:1173 http://www.aafp.org/exam.xml

[a]High risk: seeking treatment for STDs; male homosexual sex after 1975; past or present injection drug use; past or current exchange of sex for money or drugs; sex partners of people who are HIV-infected, bisexual, or injection drug users; or history of blood transfusion between 1978 and 1985.

[b]The FDA has approved 2 HIV home testing kits and warns about use of HIV home testing kits that have not been FDA approved. Consumers can obtain information about HIV home testing kits by calling the HIV/AIDS Program of the FDA in the Office of Special Health Issues at 301-827-4460. Health care provider follow-up is recommended for positive home HIV test results. [Oncology 1999;13(1):81]

HYPERTENSION, CHILDREN & ADOLESCENTS

Disease Screening	Organization	Date	Population	Recommendations	Comments	Source
Hypertension, Children & Adolescents	USPSTF	2003	Aged < 21 years	Insufficient evidence to recommend for or against routine screening	Hypertension: BP > 95th percentile 3 different times within 1 month, adjusted for height (J Pediatr 1993;123:871) (see Appendix III)	Pediatrics 1987;79:1 Pediatrics 1996;98:649
	NHLBI	1996	Aged 3–20 years	Annual screening	Major reason to screen children is early identification of conditions associated with hypertension (eg, coarctation of aorta, renal artery stenosis, renal parenchymal disease). Treatment: See footnote a.	
	Bright Futures	1994	Aged 3–21 years	Annual screening at ages 3–6, 8, and 10–21 years		
	GAPS	1994	Aged 11–18 years	Annual screening		

HYPERTENSION, ADULTS

Disease Screening	Organization	Date	Population	Recommendations	Comments	Source
Hypertension, Adults	JNC VII (NHLBI)	2003	Aged > 18 years	Annual screening If BP < 130/85 mm Hg, then every 2 years If BP 130–139/85–89 mm Hg, then annually If BP 140–159/90–99 mm Hg, then confirm within 2 months (based on JNC VI)	Prehypertension: SBP 120–139 or DBP 80–89 Stage I hypertension: SBP 140–159 or DBP 90–99 Stage II hypertension: SBP ≥ 160 or DBP ≥ 100 (based on average of ≥ 2 measurements on ≥ 2 separate office visits) Finger monitors are not accurate. [Fam Med 1996;61(50):53] Perform physical exam and routine labs.[b] Pursue secondary causes of hypertension.[c] Treatment: See footnotes d,e.	JAMA 2003;289:2560
	USPSTF	2003	Age ≥18 years	Strongly recommends screening	Ambulatory BP monitoring is a better (and independent) predictor of cardiovascular outcomes compared with office visit monitoring.	Hypertension 2000;35:844 NEJM 2003;348:2407–2415
	AAFP	2002	Aged > 21 years	"Strongly recommended" Periodic screening If BP < 140/85 mm Hg, then every 2 years If DBP 85–89 mm Hg, then annually		http://www.aafp.org/exam.xml

HYPERTENSION, ELDERLY

Disease Screening	Organization	Date	Population	Recommendations	Comments	Source
Hypertension, Elderly	JNC VI	1997	Aged > 60 years	Annual screening	Prevalence: 60%–70% of persons > 60 years old Treatment[f] (JNC VII SBP goal < 140 mm Hg)	Hypertension 1995;25:305 NEJM 1993;329:1912

[a]Treatment of primary (essential) hypertension in older children and adolescents is of unproved benefit; majority respond to weight loss and exercise. (Am J Cardiol 1983;52:763. Pediatrics 1978;61:245) The NHLBI recommends pharmacologic treatment of severe hypertension in addition to nonpharmacologic treatment (< 1% of hypertensive children are classified as severe). (Arch Dis Child 1967;42:34)

[b]Physical exam should include: measurements of height, weight, and waist circumference; funduscopic exam (retinopathy); carotid auscultation (bruit); jugular venous pulsation; thyroid gland (enlargement); cardiac auscultation (left ventricular heave, S_3 or S_4, murmurs, clicks); chest auscultation (rales, evidence of chronic obstructive pulmonary disease); abdominal exam (bruits, masses, pulsations); exam of lower extremities (diminished arterial pulsations, bruits, edema); and neurologic exam (focal findings). Routine labs include urinalysis, complete blood count, electrolytes (potassium, calcium), creatinine, glucose, fasting lipids, and 12-lead electrocardiogram.

[c]Pursue secondary causes of hypertension when evaluation is suggestive (clues in parentheses) of: (1) pheochromocytoma (labile or paroxysmal hypertension accompanied by sweats, headaches, and palpitations), (2) renovascular disease (abdominal bruits), (3) autosomal dominant polycystic kidney disease (abdominal or flank masses), (4) Cushing's syndrome (truncal obesity with purple striae), (5) primary hyperaldosteronism (hypokalemia), (6) hyperparathyroidism (hypercalcemia), (7) renal parenchymal disease (elevated serum creatinine, abnormal urinalysis), (8) poor response to drug therapy, (9) well-controlled hypertension with an abrupt increase in blood pressure, (10) SBP > 180 or DBP > 110 mm Hg, or (11) sudden onset of hypertension.

[d]Treatment goals are for BP < 140/90, unless diabetes or renal disease present (< 130/80). See JNC VII Management Algorithm, page 127.

[e]CHS/BHS pharmacologic treatment recommendations for DBP 90–99 mm Hg are dependent upon additional factors of target organ damage or diabetes. Otherwise, risk stratify according to higher pressures within the range, advanced age, male sex, smoking, dyslipidemia, or strong family history of cardiovascular disease. (BMJ 1993;306:983)

[f]Although SBP of 140–160 mm Hg is associated with greater cardiovascular morbidity, there is still no demonstration that pharmacologic therapy improves outcomes.

Disease Screening	**Organization**	**Date**	**Population**	**Recommendations**	**Comments**	**Source**
				LEAD POISONING		
Lead Poisoning	ACPM	2001	Infants and children	Selective screening at 12 months for infants and children at high risk[a]	Risk assessment should be performed during prenatal visits and continuing until 6 years of age.	Am J Prev Med 2001;20:78
	CDC AAP	2000 1998	Infants and children	Selective screening with blood lead level at 9–12 months, and again at 24 months when levels peak, of infants and children at high risk[b] Evaluation of blood lead level[c]	The Advisory Committee on Childhood Lead Poisoning Prevention (ACCLPP) includes Medicaid-enrolled children ages 1–5 years as high risk [MMWR 2000;49 (RR-14):1] CDC personal risk questionnaire: (1) Does your child live in or regularly visit a house (or other facility, eg, daycare) that was built before 1950? (2) Does your child live in or regularly visit a house built before 1978 with recent or ongoing renovations or remodeling (within the last 6 months)? (3) Does your child have a sibling or playmate who has or did have lead poisoning?	Pediatrics 1998; 101:1072 www.cdc.gov/ mmwr/pdf/rr/ rr4914.pdf
	AAFP USPSTF	2001 1996	Infants at age 12 months	Selective screening with blood lead level for those infants at high risk[d]		www.aafp.org/ exam.xml

LEAD POISONING

[a]Criteria for being at high risk include: receipt of Medicaid or WIC, living in a community with ≥ 12% prevalence of elevated blood lead levels (BLLs) at ≥ 10 µg/mL; living in a community with ≥ 27% of homes built before 1950; or meeting 1 or more high risk criteria from a lead-screening questionnaire (see CDC comments in table). Prevalence levels supported by recent cost-effectiveness studies. (Arch Pediatr Adolesc Med 1998;152:1202)

[b]High risk of lead poisoning if any one of the following conditions exists: (1) Child lives in or regularly visits a house or child care facility built before 1950; (2) child lives in or regularly visits a house or child care facility built before 1978 that is being or has recently been renovated or remodeled (within the last 6 months); or (3) child has a sibling or playmate who has or did have lead poisoning.

[c]Confirm elevated lead levels with venous sample after screening sample from fingerstick: immediately if > 70 µg/mL, within 48 hours if 45–69 µg/mL, within 1 week if 20–44 µg/mL, and within 1 month if 10–19 µg/mL. See AAP guidelines for further treatment recommendations.

[d]Increased risk of lead poisoning exists for infants who: (1) live in communities in which the prevalence of lead levels requiring intervention is high or undefined, (2) live in or frequently visit a home built before 1950 with dilapidated paint or with recent or ongoing renovation or remodeling, (3) have close contact with a person who has an elevated lead level, (4) live near lead industry or heavy traffic, or (5) live with someone whose job or hobby involves lead exposure or who uses lead-based pottery or takes traditional remedies that contain lead.

				OBESITY	
Disease Screening	Organization	Date	Population	Recommendations	Comments	Source

Disease Screening	Organization	Date	Population	Recommendations	Comments	Source
Obesity	NHLBI NIDDKD	1998	Age > 18 years	Calculate BMI for all patients. [a,b,c]	The NHLBI makes a strong case for promoting weight loss in overweight individuals, particularly those with hypertension, diabetes, cardiovascular disease, and hyperlipidemia.	NHLBI Obesity Guidelines in Adults, 1998
	AAFP Maternal and Child Health Bureau USPSTF AAP	2001 1998 1996	All age groups	Periodic height and weight measurements	Waist-hip ratio may also provide additional prognostic information beyond BMI and waist circumference. Among women 50–69 years of age free of cancer, heart disease, and diabetes, waist-hip ratio is the best anthropometric predictor of total mortality. (Arch Intern Med 2000;160:2117)	www.aafp.org/exam. xml

[a]BMI is calculated as: weight (kg)/height (m) squared. See Appendix IV for BMI Conversion Table. Overweight is defined as BMI 25–29.9 kg/m² and obesity as BMI > 30 kg/m².
[b]Studies do not support a BMI range 25–27 as a risk factor for all-cause and cardiovascular mortality among elderly (age ≥ 65 years) persons. (Arch Intern Med 2001;161:1194)
[c]BMI cut-offs may also need to be modified for some Asian populations. (www.idi.org.au; Am J Clin Nutr 2001;73:123)

Disease Screening	Organization	Date	Population	Recommendations	Comments	Source
					OSTEOPOROSIS	
Osteoporosis	ACOG NOF USPSTF AACE	2002 2002 2002 2001	Women aged ≥ 65 years	Routine screening of bone mineral density (BMD)	The benefits of screening and treatment are of at least moderate magnitude for women at ↑ risk by virtue of age or presence of other risk factors. Dual energy x-ray absorptiometry is the most accurate clinical method for identifying those with low BMD.	www.acog.org http://www.nof.org Ann Intern Med 2002; 137:526 http://www.aace.com/ clin/guidelines
	ACOG NOF USPSTF AACE American College of Rheumatology	2002 2002 2002 2001 1997	Women at increased risk for osteoporotic fractures[a]	Routine screening beginning at age 60.	The Simple Calculated Osteoporosis Risk Estimation (SCORE) and Osteoporosis Risk Assessment Instrument (ORAI) decision rules are better than NOF guidelines at targeting BMD testing in high-risk patients. (JAMA 2001;286:57–63)	www.acog.org http://www.nof.org Ann Intern Med 2002; 137:526 http://www.aace.com/ clin/guidelines www.rheumatology.org

[a]Exact risk factors that should trigger screening in this age group are difficult to specify based on evidence.
[b]High risk: chronic steroid use (≥ 2 months), repeated fractures or fractures not caused by trauma, early menopause, blood relative with osteoporosis, known low BMD, low body weight (< 127 lb), cigarette use.

OSTEOPOROSIS: SCREENING

SELECTIVE SCREENING FOR OSTEOPOROSIS IN PERSONS NOT
CURRENTLY TAKING ANTI-OSTEOPOROSIS
MEDICATIONS OR HAVING A HISTORY OF HIP FRACTURE
(Modified from the National Osteoporosis Foundation:
Physician's guide to prevention & treatment of osteoporosis;
Up To Date Screening for Osteoporosis by H.N. Rosen).

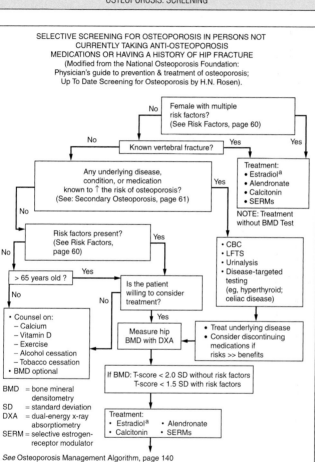

BMD = bone mineral
densitometry
SD = standard deviation
DXA = dual-energy x-ray
absorptiometry
SERM = selective estrogen-
receptor modulator

See Osteoporosis Management Algorithm, page 140

[a]*See* data alert regarding HRT, page 124.

RISK FACTORS FOR OSTEOPOROTIC FRACTURE	
Potentially Modifiable	**Nonmodifiable**
Current cigarette smoker	*Personal history of fracture as an adult*
Low body weight (< 127 lb)	*History of fracture in first-degree relative*
Estrogen deficiency: -early menopause (age < 45 years) or bilateral ovariectomy -prolonged premenopausal amenorrhea (> 1 year)	Caucasian race
Low calcium intake (lifelong)	Advanced age
Alcohol (> 2 drinks/day)	Female sex
Impaired eyesight despite adequate correction	Dementia
Recurrent falls	
Inadequate physical activity	
Poor health/frailty	

Italicized items—personal or family history of fracture, smoking, and low body weight—were demonstrated in a large, ongoing, prospective U.S. study to be key factors in determining the risk of hip fracture (independent of bone density).

Source: National Osteoporosis Foundation.

Physician's guide to prevention and treatment of osteoporosis. Available at: http://www.nof.org/physguide/ Accessed December 12, 2003.

CAUSES OF GENERALIZED SECONDARY OSTEOPOROSIS IN ADULTS

Drugs	Endocrine Diseases or Metabolic Causes	Collagen-Vascular Diseases	Nutritional Conditions	Other Causes
Aluminum	Acromegaly	Epidermolysis bullosa	Gastrectomy	Amyloidosis
Anticonvulsants	Adrenal atrophy and	Osteogenesis	Eating	Ankylosing
Cigarette smoking	Addison's disease	imperfecia	disorders	spondylitis
Cytotoxic drugs	Congenital porphyria		Malabsorption	AIDS/HIV
Excessive alcohol	Cushing's syndrome		syndromes	Chronic
Excessive thyroxine	Endometriosis		Nutritional	obstructive
Glucocorticosteroids &	Female athlete triad		disorders	pulmonary
adrenocorticotropin	Gaucher's disease		Parenteral	disease
(oral or inhaled)	Gonadal insufficiency		nutrition	Hemophilia
Gonadotropin-	(primary &		Pernicious	Idiopathic
releasing hormone	secondary)		anemia	scoliosis
agonists	Hemochromatosis		Severe liver	Inflammatory
Heparin	Hyperparathyroidism		disease	bowel
Immune suppressants	Hypophosphatemia		(especially	disease
Lithium	Diabetes mellitus		primary	Lymphoma &
Tamoxifen	type 1		biliary	leukemia
(premenopausal use)	Thyrotoxicosis		cirrhosis)	Mastocytosis
	Tumor secretion of		Sprue	Multiple
	parathyroid			myeloma
	hormone–related			Multiple
	peptide			sclerosis
				Rheumatoid
				arthritis
				Sarcoidosis
				Spinal cord
				transection
				Stroke
				Thalassemia

Source: National Osteoporosis Foundation.
Physician's guide to prevention and treatment of osteoporosis. Available at:
http://www.nof.org/physguide/ Accessed December 12, 2003.

Disease Screening	Organization	Date	Population	Recommendations	Comments	Source
SCOLIOSIS						
Scoliosis	Bright Futures	2002	Adolescents	Screen during physical exam annually in adolescents and children > 8 years of age.		
	USPSTF CTF	1996 1994	Adolescents	Insufficient evidence to recommend for or against routine screening of asymptomatic adolescents.	Positive predictive value of bending test is 42.8% for scoliosis of > 5 degrees and 6.4% for > 15 degrees; sensitivity 74%, specificity 78%. (Am J Public Health 1985;75:1377)	
	AAOS	1992	Adolescents	Screen girls twice (ages 10 and 12 years) and boys once (age 13 or 14 years).		www.aaos.org
	Scoliosis Research Society	1986	Adolescents	Perform annual screening of all children ages 10–14 years.		Scoliosis Research Society: Scoliosis: A Handbook for Patients. Scoliosis Research Society, 1986

	SYPHILIS				
Disease Screening	Organization	Date	Population	Recommendations	Comments	Source

Disease Screening	Organization	Date	Population	Recommendations	Comments	Source
Syphilis	AAFP AAP & ACOG USPSTF	2002 1997 1996	Pregnant women and high-risk persons[a,b]	Screen all pregnant women with nontreponemal test (eg, RPR or VDRL) at first prenatal visit; repeat in third trimester and at delivery for women at high risk of acquiring infection during pregnancy. Screen high-risk (nonpregnant) persons with routine serologic test (nontreponemal test; eg, RPR or VDRL).	All reactive nontreponemal tests should be confirmed with a more specific treponemal test (eg, FTA-ABS). Perform follow-up serologic tests after treatment to document decline in titers (using the same test used initially). Sensitivity of nontreponemal tests varies with levels of antibodies: 62%–76% in early primary syphilis, 100% during secondary syphilis, and 70% in untreated late syphilis. In late syphilis, previously reactive results revert to nonreactive in 25% of patients. Specificity of nontreponemal tests is 75%–85% in persons with preexisting diseases or conditions (eg, collagen vascular diseases, injection drug use, advanced malignancy, pregnancy, malaria, tuberculosis, viral and rickettsial diseases) and 100% in persons without preexisting diseases or conditions. Syphilis outbreaks have been recently reported among California gay men and Alabama prisoners. (Am J Public Health 2001;91:1220, JAMA 2001;285:1285)	Ann Intern Med 1986;104:368 Pediatrics 1994;94:568 MMWR 1993;42 (RR-14):1 http://www.aafp.org/exam.xml

[a]High risk includes commercial sex workers, persons who exchange sex for money or drugs, persons with other STDs (including HIV), and sexual contacts of persons with active syphilis.

[b]The American Academy of Neurology does not recommend syphilis screening in persons with dementia unless clinical suspicion for neurosyphilis is present. (Neurology 2001;56:1143)

						THYROID DISEASE
Disease Screening	Organization	Date	Population	Recommendations	Comments	Source
Thyroid Disease	AAFP USPSTF	2002 1996	Children and adults	Routine screening is not recommended.	Increased risk of hypothyroidism among patients with autoimmune diseases, unexplained depression, cognitive dysfunction, or hypercholesterolemia.	www.aafp.org/exam. xml
	ATA	2000	Women aged ≥ 35 years	Screen with serum TSH at age 35 years, and every 5 years thereafter.	Individuals with symptoms and signs potentially attributable to thyroid dysfunction[a] and those with risk factors for its development[b] may require more frequent TSH testing. When there is suspicion of pituitary or hypothalamic disease, the serum FT4 concentration should be measured in addition to the serum TSH.	Arch Intern Med 2000;160:1573
	ACP	1998	Women aged > 50 years	Perform selective screening for women with 1 or more general symptoms such as fatigue, weight gain, or depression.		Ann Intern Med 1998;129:141–143
	USPSTF	1996	Elderly	Insufficient evidence to recommend for or against screening.	Clinicians should remain alert for subtle or nonspecific symptoms of hypothyroidism and maintain a low threshold for diagnostic evaluation using serum TSH. Controversy exists regarding Rx benefit for patients with subclinical hypothyroidism (elevated TSH; normal free thyroxine).	NEJM 2001;345(4): 260–264. J Gen Intern Med 1996;11:744 Ann Intern Med 1984;101:18

THYROID DISEASE

Disease Screening	Organization	Date	Population	Recommendations	Comments	Source
Thyroid Disease (continued)	AACE	2002	Elderly	Periodic screening with sensitive TSH		www.aace.com/clin/ guidelines Endocrine Practice 2002;8:457–469

[a]Signs, symptoms, and comorbidities suggestive of hypothyroidism include previous thyroid dysfunction; goiter; surgery or radiotherapy affecting the thyroid; diabetes mellitus; vitiligo; pernicious anemia; leukotrichia (prematurely gray hair); and medications (such as lithium carbonate and iodine-containing compounds, eg, amiodarone, radiocontrast agents, expectorants containing potassium iodide, and kelp).

[b]Risk factors include family history of thyroid disease, or personal history of pernicious anemia, diabetes mellitus, and primary adrenal insufficiency. Laboratory test results suggestive of thyroid disease include hypercholesterolemia, hyponatremia, anemia, CPK and LDH elevations, hyperprolactinemia, hypercalcemia, alkaline phosphatase elevation, and hepatocellular enzyme elevation.

	TUBERCULOSIS					
Disease Screening	Organization	Date	Population	Recommendations	Comments	Source
Tuberculosis	CDC AAFP Bright Futures ATS USPSTF AAP CTF	2003 2002 2002 2001 1996 1994 1994	Persons at increased risk of developing TB[a]	Screening by tuberculin skin test is recommended. Frequency of testing should be based on likelihood of further exposure to TB and level of confidence in the accuracy of the results.[b,c]	Persons with positive PPD test should receive chest x-ray and clinical evaluation for TB. If no evidence of active infection, provide INH prophylaxis if appropriate. The purpose of targeted testing is to find and treat persons who have both latent TB infection and high risk for TB disease. Persons at low risk for developing TB and who have had a skin test for other reasons (such as baseline PPD of health care workers) are not necessarily candidates for treatment if found to be infected. (Am J Resp Crit Care Med 2000;161:S221) Treatment (INH for 9 months) is recommended for foreign-born persons from countries with a high prevalence of TB who have latent TB infection and who have been in the United States < 5 years. Because sporadic severe INH-associated liver injury still occurs, patients taking INH should be monitored as indicated (history of liver disorder, HIV infection, pregnant and immediate post-partum women, regular alcohol user). [MMWR 2001;50(34)] QuantiFERON-TB (QTF) may be considered in selected populations. [MMWR 2003;52(RR-02):15–18]	Pediatrics 1994;93:131 www.aafp.org/exam.xml Am Rev Respir Dis 1992;146:1623 Pediatrics 1996;97:282 MMWR 2003;52(RR-02):15–18 MMWR 2000;49(RR-06):1–54

TUBERCULOSIS

[a]Increased risk: persons infected with HIV, close contacts of persons with known or suspected TB (including health care workers), persons with medical risk factors associated with reactivation of TB (eg, silicosis, diabetes mellitus, prolonged corticosteroid therapy, immunosuppressive therapy), end-stage renal disease, immunosuppressive therapy), immigrants from countries with high TB prevalence (eg, most countries in Africa, Asia, and Latin America), medically underserved and low-income populations, alcoholics, injection drug users, persons with abnormal CXRs compatible with past TB, and residents of long-term care facilities (eg, correctional institutions, mental institutions, nursing homes).

[b]Periodic (eg, ages 1, 4–6, and 6–11 years) tuberculin skin testing is recommended for children who live in high-prevalence regions or whose history for risk factors is incomplete or unreliable.

[c]Test: Give intradermal injection of 5 U of tuberculin PPD and examine 48–72 hours later. Criteria for positive skin test (diameter of induration): > 15 mm for low risk, > 10 mm for high risk (including children < 4 years of age), > 5 mm for very high risk (HIV, abnormal CXR, recent contact with infected persons). If negative, consider 2-step testing to differentiate between booster effect and new conversion. Perform second test within 13 weeks. False-negative results occur in 5%–10%, especially early in infection, with anergy, with concurrent severe illness, in newborns and infants < 3 months old, and with improper technique. Prior BCG vaccination is not considered a valid basis for dismissing positive results.

	VISUAL IMPAIRMENT, GLAUCOMA, & CATARACTS				
Disease Screening	Organization	Date	Population	Recommendations	Comments	Source
Visual Impairment, Glaucoma, & Cataracts	AAO AOA AAP Bright Futures	1997 1997 1996 1994	Infants and children	Eye and vision screening is recommended between birth and 2 months, at age 6 months, ages 3–5 years, and ages 5–6 years. AOA recommends continuing comprehensive eye and vision exams every 2 years thereafter.		www.aao.org www.aoanet.org Pediatrics 1996;98:153
	AAFP USPSTF	2002 1996	Children	AAFP: "Recommends" Vision screening for amblyopia and strabismus for all children once before entering school, preferably between ages 3 and 4 years. Insufficient evidence to recommend for or against routine screening for decreased visual acuity among asymptomatic school children.		www.aafp.org/exam.xml
	USPSTF	1996	Adults	Insufficient evidence to recommend for or against routine eye and vision screening among asymptomatic nonelderly adults. Insufficient evidence to recommend for or against routine screening for elevated intraocular pressure or glaucoma by primary care physicians.		

VISUAL IMPAIRMENT, GLAUCOMA, & CATARACTS

Disease Screening	Organization	Date	Population	Recommendations	Comments	Source
Visual Impairment, Glaucoma, & Cataracts (continued)	AAO	2000	Adults	Comprehensive eye and vision exam every 3–5 years in blacks aged 20–39 years, and, regardless of race, every 2–4 years aged 40–64 years and every 1–2 years beginning age 65 years.		www.aao.org
	AOA	1997	Adults	Comprehensive eye and vision exam every 2–3 years aged 18–40 years, every 2 years aged 41–60 years, and every 1 year aged ≥ 61 years		www.aoanet.org
	AAFP AGS USPSTF	2001 1997 1996	Elderly	Perform routine eye and Snellen visual acuity screening. Optimal frequency is not known.		J Am Geriatr Soc 1997;45:344 http://www.aafp.org/exam.xml

2
Disease Prevention

Disease	Organization	Date	Population	Recommendations	Comments	Source
BREAST CANCER						
Breast Cancer	NCI	2002	Women	Avoid unnecessary breast irradiation. Low-fat diet and exercise may decrease risk. Alcohol may increase risk. <u>Genetic Screening:</u> Little evidence to support or quantify potential beneficial effect of genetic screening (*BRCA1/BRCA2*). <u>Tamoxifen:</u> Risks and benefits have to be weighed, and decisions regarding use of tamoxifen for prevention must be individualized. <u>Mastectomy:</u> Because of the physical and psychological effects and the irreversibility of the procedure, decisions regarding this option must be considered on an individual basis.	Known genetic syndromes contribute to ~5% of breast cancers. An RCT has shown that tamoxifen reduces the risk of developing breast cancer in women at increased risk. Tamoxifen increases the risk of endometrial cancer and of thrombotic vascular events. (*J Natl Cancer Inst* 1998;90:1371) Bilateral prophylactic mastectomy is associated with a reduction in risk of breast cancer by as much as 90% among women with an increased risk of breast cancer due to a strong family history or with BRCA1 or BRCA2 alterations.	www.cancer.gov J Natl Cancer Inst 2001; 93(21):1633–1637 NEJM 1999;340(2): 77–84
	CTF	2000	Low-/normal-risk women (< 1.66% on Gail index)[a]	Recommend against use of tamoxifen to reduce the risk of breast cancer.		

						BREAST CANCER		

Disease	Organization	Date	Population	Recommendations	Comments	Source
Breast Cancer (continued)	ASCO CTF	2002 2001	Women at high risk[a]	For women with a 5-year projected risk of breast cancer of $\geq 1.66\%$, tamoxifen (at 20 mg/day for up to 5 years) may be offered to reduce their risk. Tamoxifen use should be discussed as part of an informed decision-making process, with careful consideration of risks and benefits. Premature to recommend raloxifene, tamoxifen combined with hormone replacement therapy, aromatase inhibitors or inactivators, or fenretinide use to lower the risk of developing breast cancer outside of a clinical trial setting.[b]	Women being considered for tamoxifen therapy should be evaluated by health care providers familiar with evaluation of individual breast cancer risk and the risks and benefits of tamoxifen use.	www.asco.org J Clin Oncol 1999;17(6):1939 CMAJ 2001; 164(12):1681–1690

[a]Predicted risk of breast cancer calculated by using the Gail model, which considers age, number of first-degree relatives with breast cancer, number of previous breast biopsies, age at first live birth, and age at menarche. (J Natl Cancer Inst 1999;91:1829) The Breast Cancer Risk Assessment Tool allows health professionals to project a woman's individualized estimate of risk for invasive breast cancer over a 5-year period and lifetime. (http://bcra.nci.nih.gov/brc)

[b]Among postmenopausal women with osteoporosis, the risk of invasive breast cancer was decreased by 75% during 3 years of treatment with raloxifene. [JAMA 1999;281(23):2189] The MORE trial found that measurement of estradiol level by sensitive assay in postmenopausal women identifies those at high risk of breast cancer. These women benefited most from reduction in risk of breast cancer with raloxifene treatment. (JAMA 2002;287:216–220) The Study of Tamoxifen and Raloxifene (STAR) began recruiting volunteers in May 1999. This study will compare tamoxifen and raloxifene for their effects on reduction of breast cancer development in postmenopausal women. Information about this and other breast cancer prevention trials is available from http://cancer.gov/star or from the National Cancer Institute's Cancer Information Service (1-800-422-6237). The NCI is conducting the Capital Area SERM study to evaluate the safety of raloxifene in premenopausal women who are at increased risk for breast cancer (1-888-624-1937).

	DIABETES, TYPE 2				
Disease	Organization	Date	Population	Recommendations	Comments
Diabetes (Type 2)	ADA	2003	Patients identified through screening with impaired fasting glucose or glucose tolerance (see page 42).	Counsel on increasing physical activity and weight loss. Follow-up counseling important for success. Monitor for diabetes every 1–2 years.	Drug therapy should not be routinely used to prevent diabetes until more information is known about cost-effectiveness. RCTs have proven the efficacy of increased physical activity and weight loss for preventing Type 2 diabetes. (NEJM 2002;346:393) In overweight patients (mean BMI, 34 kg/m^2), nutrition/exercise intervention group had 4.8% incidence of progression to diabetes compared with control group (11.0% incidence).

Source: Diabetes Care 2003;26(Suppl 1): S62

Disease	Organization	Date	Population	Recommendations	Comments	Source
ENDOCARDITIS						
Endocarditis	ASCRS	2000	High-risk persons[a]	Give antibiotic prophylaxis[c] before bacteremia-producing procedures.[d,e]		JAMA 1997;277:1794
	AHA	1997	Moderate-risk persons[b]			

[a]Patients at high risk for endocarditis include those with prosthetic heart valves (including bioprosthetic and homograft valves), previous bacterial endocarditis, complex cyanotic congenital heart disease (including single ventricle states, transposition of the great arteries, tetralogy of Fallot), and surgically constructed systemic pulmonary shunts or conduits.

[b]Patients at moderate risk for endocarditis include those with most other congenital heart diseases (excluding isolated secundum atrial septal defect and surgically repaired atrial septal defect, ventricular septal defect, or patent ductus arteriosus without residua beyond 6 months), acquired valvular dysfunction (eg, rheumatic heart disease), hypertrophic cardiomyopathy, and mitral valve prolapse with valvular regurgitation or thickened leaflets.

[c]Standard prophylaxis regimen for dental, oral, respiratory tract, or esophageal procedures: amoxicillin (adults 2.0 g; children 50 mg/kg orally 1 hour before procedure). If unable to take oral medications, give ampicillin (adults 2.0 g IM or IV; children 50 mg/kg IM or IV within 30 minutes of procedure). If penicillin-allergic, give clindamycin (adults 600 mg; children 20 mg/kg orally 1 hour before procedure) or cephalexin or cefadroxil (adults 2.0 g; children 50 mg/kg orally 1 hour before procedure), or azithromycin or clarithromycin (adults 500 mg; children 15 mg/kg orally 1 hour before procedure). If penicillin-allergic and unable to take oral medications, give clindamycin (adults 600 mg; children 20 mg/kg IV within 30 minutes before procedure) or cefazolin (adults 1 g; children 25 mg/kg IM or IV within 30 minutes of procedure). See reference for recommended antibiotic regimens for other procedures. (JAMA 1997;277:1794)

[d]Bacteremia-producing procedures include: (1) dental and oral procedures including dental extractions, periodontal procedures, dental implant placement and reimplantation of avulsed teeth, endodontic (root canal) instrumentation, subgingival placement of antibiotic fibers or strips, initial placement of orthodontic bands but not brackets, intraligamentary local anesthetic injections, and prophylactic cleaning of teeth or implants where bleeding is anticipated; (2) respiratory tract procedures including tonsillectomy and adenoidectomy, surgical operations involving the respiratory mucosa, and bronchoscopy with a rigid bronchoscope; and (3) genitourinary tract procedures including prostatic surgery, cystoscopy, and urethral dilation.

[e]Prophylaxis for high-risk but not moderate-risk patients is recommended for patients undergoing gastrointestinal tract procedures including sclerotherapy, esophageal stricture dilation, ERCP with biliary obstruction, biliary tract surgery, surgical operations involving the intestinal mucosa, and colon and rectal endoscopy. (Dis Colon Rectum 2000;43:1193)

FALLS IN THE ELDERLY

Older person who:
- Presents for medical attention due to a fall, or
- Reports ≥ 1 fall in past year, or
- Demonstrates abnormalities of gait and/or balance

↓

Fall evaluation:
- History: fall circumstances, medications, acute or chronic medical problems, mobility
- Exam: vision, gait and balance, lower extremity joint function, neurologic function (mental status; muscle strength; lower extremity peripheral nerves; proprioception; reflexes; cortical, extrapyramidal, and cerebellar function), cardiovascular status (heart rate and rhythm, postural pulse and blood pressure, heart rate and blood pressure response to carotid sinus stimulation)

↓

Multifactorial interventions:
(as appropriate, based on evaluation)
- Appropriate use of assistive devices
- Exercise programs, with balance training
- Gait training
- Modification of environmental hazards
- Review and modification of medications, especially psychotropics
- Staff education at long-term care and assisted-living settings
- Treatment of cardiovascular disorders
- Treatment of postural hypotension

Source: JAGS 2001;49:664–672 and NEJM 2003;348:42–49.

	HYPERTENSION				

Disease	Organization	Date	Population	Recommendations	Comments	Source
Hyper-tension	NHLBI	2002	Persons at risk for developing hypertension[a]	Recommend weight loss, reduced sodium intake, moderate alcohol consumption, increased physical activity, potassium supplementation, modification of eating patterns (see Lifestyle Modifications for Primary Prevention of Hypertension).	A 2-mm Hg reduction in the population average of diastolic BP for white U.S. residents 35–64 years of age would result in a 17% decrease in hypertension, a 14% reduction in stroke risk, and a 6% reduction in heart disease risk. (Arch Intern Med 1995;155:701)	JAMA 2002:288: 1882

[a]Family history of hypertension, African-American (black race) ancestry, overweight or obesity, sedentary lifestyle, excess intake of dietary sodium, insufficient intake of potassium, excess consumption of alcohol.

LIFESTYLE MODIFICATIONS FOR PRIMARY PREVENTION OF HYPERTENSION

- Maintain normal body weight for adults (BMI, 18.5–24.9 kg/m^2)
- Reduce dietary sodium intake to no more than 100 mmol/d (approximately 6 g of sodium chloride or 2.4 g of sodium/day)
- Engage in regular aerobic physical activity such as brisk walking (at least 30 minutes/day, most days of the week)
- Limit alcohol consumption to no more than 1 oz (30 mL) of ethanol [e.g., 24 oz (720 mL) of beer, 10 oz (300 mL) of wine, or 2 oz (60 mL) of 100-proof whiskey] per day in most men and to no more than 0.5 oz [15 mL] of ethanol per day in women and lighter-weight persons
- Maintain adequate intake of dietary potassium [> 90 mmol (3,500 mg)/day]
- Consume a diet that is rich in fruits and vegetables and in low-fat dairy products with a reduced content of saturated and total fat [Dietary Approaches to Stop Hypertension (DASH) eating plan]

	MYOCARDIAL INFARCTION				
Disease	Organization	Date	Population	Recommendations	Comments	Source
Myocardial Infarction	AHA	2002	All	Begin risk factor assessment at age 20 years. <u>Dietary guidelines:</u> (1) Match energy intake with energy needs. (2) Reduce saturated fat (< 10% calories), cholesterol (< 300 mg/day), and trans-fatty acids by substituting grains and unsaturated fatty acids. (3) Limit salt intake (< 6 g/day). (4) Limit alcohol (≤ 2 drinks/day in men; ≤ 1 drink per day in women). <u>Physical activity:</u> ≥ 30 minutes of moderate intensity (15–20 minutes/mile) for most days of week. <u>Control weight:</u> achieve and maintain BMI at 18.5–24.9 kg/m^2 (see Appendix IV). Strongly encourage <u>smoking cessation.</u>	Based on the Nurses' Health Study, women adhering to all 4 recommendations had a relative risk of coronary events of 0.17 compared to all other women. (NEJM 2000;343:16)	Circulation 2002;106:388 Circulation 2000;102:2284
	AHA NCEP III	2002 2002	Hyperlipidemia[a]	For screening recommendations, see page 36; also see NCEP III screening and management (page 131) recommendations.	Short-term reduction in LDL using dietary counseling by dietitians is superior to that achieved by physicians. (Am J Med 2000;109:549)	Circulation 2002;106:338
	JNC VII	2003	Hypertension	See page 127 for JNC VII treatment algorithms.	Meta-analysis suggests that beta-blockers should not be first-line therapy for uncomplicated hypertension in persons aged > 60 years. (JAMA 1998;279:1903)	

Disease	Organization	Date	Population	Recommendations	Comments	Source
Myocardial Infarction (continued)	AHA	2002	Hypertension	Goal: < 140/90; < 130/85 if renal insufficiency or heart failure present; < 130/80 if diabetes present.		Circulation 2002;106:388
	AHA	2002	Diabetes	Goals: normal fasting glucose (< 110 mg/dL) and near normal HbA1c (< 7%).	ACE inhibitors should be first choice for diabetics with hypertension. (NEJM 1998;338:645, BMJ 1998;317:703, Diabetes Care 1998;21:597), and may be superior in reducing risk for acute MI, but not stroke. (Diabetes Care 2000;23:888, J Hypertens 2000;18:1671) Studies are supporting more aggressive BP control in this population (eg, < 130/80 mm Hg). (Lancet 1998;351:1755)	Circulation 2002;106:388

<table>
<tr><td>[a]RCTs have demonstrated the CHD and mortality benefit and safety of treatment of patients with hypercholesterolemia (pravastatin, 40 mg/day) (NEJM 1995;333:1301) and the CHD benefit of treatment of average cholesterol and LDL levels (but low HDL) (lovastatin, 20–40 mg/d). (JAMA 1998;279:1615)</td></tr>
</table>

	OSTEOPOROSIS				
Disease	Organization	Date	Population	Recommendations	Comments	Source
Osteoporosis	ACOG AAFP NOF AACE NIH USPSTF CTF	2003 2002 2002 2001 2001 1996 1994	Women[b]	Counsel all women about fracture risk reduction (dietary calcium, vitamin D, weight-bearing exercise, smoking cessation, moderate alcohol intake).[a] Predictors of low bone mass include increased age, estrogen deficiency, white race, low weight and BMI, family history of osteoporosis, smoking, history of prior fractures, oral or inhaled glucocorticoid therapy use.[c] Use of alcohol and caffeine-containing beverages is inconsistently associated with decreased bone mass. Grip strength and current exercise are associated with increased bone mass. Hormone therapy: Women's Health Initiative found that use of conjugated equine estrogen (0.625 mg/day) and medroxyprogesterone acetate (2.5 mg/day) reduced the risk of hip fracture by 33%. The change in bone mineral density after 3 years was 4.5% higher for lumbar spine and 3.6% higher for total hip for hormone users vs. non-users. (JAMA 2003;290:1729–1748) ACOG continues to support the judicious, individualized use of estrogen and progestin for bone protection (www.acog.org).	Medical disorders associated with osteoporosis include hypogonadism (men),[d] use of glucocorticoids, thyroid hormone excess, anticonvulsant therapy, hypercalciuria, hyperparathyroidism, and malabsorption.	www.acog.org http://www.aafp.org/ http://www.nof.org JAMA 2001;285: 785–795 Endocrine Practice 2001;4:293–312 NEJM 2001;345: 941–947; 989–992

				OSTEOPOROSIS		
Disease	Organization	Date	Population	Recommendations	Comments	Source
Osteoporosis (continued)				Alendronate: Approved for prevention of bone loss in recently menopausal women and treatment of established osteoporosis in men and women. Has been shown to increase BMD by 5%–10% and to decrease fracture incidence by 50%. Recommended dose: 5 mg per day (35 mg per week) for recently menopausal women; 10 mg per day (70 mg per week) for established osteoporosis. Treatment efficacy demonstrated for 7 years. Risedronate: Approved for prevention and treatment of postmenopausal and glucocorticoid-induced osteoporosis. Has been shown to increase BMD and decrease fracture incidence by 30%–50%. Recommended dose 5 mg per day. Raloxifene: Approved for prevention and treatment of postmenopausal osteoporosis. Has been shown to decrease the risk of vertebral fracture by 50% and to increase BMD. Recommended dosing: 60 mg per day. Statins: Statin use did not improve fracture risk or bone density in the Women's Health Initiative Observational Study. (Ann Intern Med 2003;139:97–104)		

[a] Recommended calcium: 9–18 years, 1,300 mg/d; 19–50 years, 1,000 mg/d; > 50 years, 1,200 mg/d. Recommended vitamin D: 400–800 IU/day.

[b] For women receiving thyroid replacement therapy for nonmalignant conditions, periodically monitor and adjust dose.

[c] Consider bisphosphonate (alendronate or risedronate) for all adult women who require > 7.5 mg prednisone (or equivalent) for > 3 weeks.

[d] Early evidence indicates that testosterone replacement therapy may enhance bone mass in hypogonadal men; longer-term studies are needed to better define risks and benefits. (JAGS 2001;49:179–187)

OSTEOPOROSIS: PREVENTION FOR WOMEN AT RISK*

1. <u>COUNSEL ON:</u>
   - Tobacco cessation
   - Limit alcohol intake
   - Regular weight-bearing exercise ≥ 30 min. 3x/wk
     Muscle strengthening exercise
   - Adequate Ca^{2+} intake 1,000–1,200 mg/day
     Adequate vitamin D 800 IU/day

2. <u>IDENTIFY AND REMEDY SECONDARY CAUSES</u>
   (see table, page 61)

PERIMENOPAUSAL/POSTMENOPAUSAL

- Identify and treat sensory deficits, neurologic disease & arthritis, all of which can lead to ↑ frequency of falls
- Adjust drug dosages for drugs that are sedating, slow reflexes, ↓ coordination & impairing a person's ability to break impact of a fall
- Gait & balance training to ↓ risk of falls
- Identify and treat ♀ with osteoporosis-related fractures and those with low bone mass.

ELDERLY

- See perimenopausal/postmenopausal recommendations; in addition:
- Anchor rugs
- Minimize clutter
- Remove loose wires
- Use non-skid mats
- Add handrails in halls, bathrooms, & stairwells
- Ensure adequate lighting in halls, stairwells, & entrances
- Wear sturdy low-heeled shoes

Source: Adapted from AACE clinical practice guidelines for the prevention & treatment of postmenopausal osteoporosis.

*See page 60 for description of risks.

Disease	Organization	Date	Population	Recommendations	Comments	Source
				STROKE		
Stroke	JNC VII AHA	2003 2002	Hypertension	See Myocardial Infarction, pages 79–80.		Circulation 2002;106:388
	AHA	2002	Atrial fibrillation	Goal: normal sinus rhythm or, if chronic atrial fibrillation, anticoagulation with INR 2.0–3.0 (target, 2.5). Aged < 65 years, no risk factors: aspirin Aged < 65 years, w/risk factors:[a] warfarin (INR 2.0–3.0) Aged 65–75 years, no risk factors: aspirin or warfarin Aged 65–75 years w/risk factors: warfarin (INR 2.0–3.0) Aged > 75 years: warfarin (INR 2.0–3.0) See pages 109–110 for atrial fibrillation management algorithm.	Average stroke rate in patients with risk factors about 5% per year (in those with no hx of stroke or TIA). Meta-analysis concluded that adjusted-dose warfarin reduced the absolute risk of stroke by about 2.7% per year (NNT = 37) compared with 1.5% reduction for aspirin (NNT = 67). Risk of major bleed = 0.6% per year (NNH = 167); risk of intracranial bleed = 0.3% per year (NNH = 333). (Ann Intern Med 1999;131:492).	Circulation 2002;106:388 Circulation 2001;103:163
	ACCP	2001	Atrial fibrillation	Give anticoagulation with warfarin; target prothrombin time INR = 2.5 (range, 2.0–3.0). All patients with any high risk factor for stroke[b] or > 1 moderate risk factor for stroke[c]: Give warfarin as above. Patients with 1 moderate risk factor[c]: Give aspirin or oral anticoagulants. Patients with no high or moderate risk factors: Give aspirin, 325 mg/day.	For mechanical heart valve recommendations, see Chest 2001;119(1 Suppl):220S–227S.	Chest 2001;119(1 Suppl):194S

STROKE					
Disease	**Organization**	**Date**	**Population**	**Recommendations**	**Comments**	**Source**

Disease	Organization	Date	Population	Recommendations	Comments	Source
Stroke (continued)	ACP	1994	Atrial fibrillation	Similar to ACCP, except uses age 60 years as cutoff for no risk factors.		Ann Intern Med 1994;121:54
	AHA	2002	Diabetes	See Myocardial Infarction, pages 79–80.		Circulation 2002;106:388
	AHA CNS USPSTF	2001 1997 1996	Carotid artery stenosis	See page 31 for screening and treatment guidelines. Clear consensus exists on efficacy of treatment for symptomatic CAS; treatment of asymptomatic CAS is controversial.		Circulation 2001;103:163 CMAJ 1997;157:653 J Vasc Surg 1992;15:469
	AHA	2002	Hyperlipidemia	See screening recommendations on page 36. See Myocardial Infarction, pages 79–80.		Circulation 2002;106:388
	AHA	2002	Smoking	Strongly encourage patient and family to stop smoking. Provide counseling, nicotine replacement, and formal programs as available.		Circulation 2002;106:388

[a]Atrial fibrillation risk factors: hypertension, diabetes mellitus, poor left ventricular function, rheumatic mitral valve disease, prior TIA/stroke, systemic embolism or stroke, prosthetic heart valve (may require higher target INR).
[b]High risk factors for stroke in patients with atrial fibrillation include previous transient ischemic attack or stroke or embolus, hypertension, poor LV function, age > 75 years, diabetes, rheumatic mitral valve disease, and prosthetic heart valves.
[c]Moderate risk factors for stroke are age 65–75 years, diabetes, and coronary artery disease with preserved LV function.

RECOMMENDED CHILDHOOD IMMUNIZATION SCHEDULE (ACIP, AAP, AAFP)

Vaccine	Birth	1 mo	2 mo	4 mo	6 mo	12 mo	15 mo	18 mo	24 mo	4–6 y	11–12 y	14–18 y
HBV[b]	Hep B 1	only if mother HBs Ag(−) / Hep B #2			Hep B #3				Hep B[c] series			
DTaP[d]			DTaP	DTaP	DTaP		DTaP[d]			DTaP	Td	
Hib[e]			Hib	Hib	Hib	Hib						
Inactivated polio virus			IPV	IPV	IPV					IPV		
Pneumococcal conjugate[f]			PCV	PCV	PCV		PCV		PCV		PPV	
MMR[g]						MMR #1				MMR #2	MMR[c] #2	
Varicella[h]						Var					Var[c]	
HAV[i]										Hep A series		
Influenza[j]					For high risk[j] (yearly)							

Age[a]

☐ Range of acceptable ages for vaccination. Any dose not given at the recommended age should be given as a "catch-up" immunization at any subsequent visit when indicated and feasible.

[a]This schedule indicates the recommended ages for routine administration of currently licensed childhood vaccines, as of 12/1/02. Additional vaccines may be licensed and recommended during the year. Licensed combination vaccines may be used whenever any components of the combination are indicated and its other components are not contraindicated. Providers should consult the manufacturers' package inserts for detailed recommendations.

[b]All infants should receive the first dose of hepatitis B vaccine soon after birth and before hospital discharge; the first dose may be given by age 2 months if the mother is HBs Ag-negative. Only monovalent hepatitis B vaccine can be used for the birth dose. Monovalent or combination vaccine containing hepatitis B may be used to complete the series. The second dose should be given at least 4 weeks after the first, except for combination vaccines which cannot be administered before age 6 weeks. The third dose should be administered at least 16 weeks after the first dose and at least 8 weeks after the second dose, but not before age 6 months. Infants of HBsAg-positive mothers: should receive hepatitis B vaccine and 0.5 mL hepatitis B immune globulin (HBIG) within 12 hours of birth at separate sites. The second dose is recommended at 1–2 months of age, and the third dose at age 6 months. These infants should be tested for HBsAg and anti-HBs at 9–15 months of age. Infants for whom maternal HBsAg status is unknown: should receive hepatitis B vaccine within 12 hours of birth. Maternal blood should be drawn as soon as possible to determine maternal HBsAg status; if the HBsAg is positive, the infant should receive hepatitis B immune globulin as soon as possible (no later than age 1 week). The second dose is recommended at 1–2 months of age, and the third dose at age 6 months. All children and adolescents (through age 18 years) who have not been vaccinated against hepatitis B may begin the series during any visit. Special efforts should be made to vaccinate children who were born in or whose parents were born in areas of the world where HBV infection is moderately or highly endemic.

[c]Vaccines to be assessed and administered if necessary.

[d]The fourth dose of DTaP (diphtheria and tetanus toxoids and acellular pertussis vaccine) may be administered as early as age 12 months, provided 6 months have elapsed since the third dose, particularly if the child is unlikely to return at ages 15–18 months. Td (tetanus and diphtheria toxoids) is recommended at ages 11–12 years if at least 5 years have elapsed since the last dose of DTP, DTaP, or DT. Subsequent routine Td boosters are recommended every 10 years.

[e]Three Haemophilus influenzae type b (Hib) conjugate vaccines are licensed for infant use. If PRP-OMP (PedvaxHIB® or ComVax®) is administered at ages 2 and 4 months, a dose at age 6 months is not required. DTaP/Hib combination products should not be used for primary immunization in infants at 2, 4, or 6 months of age, but can be used for boosters following any Hib vaccine.

[f]The heptavalent conjugate pneumococcal vaccine (PCV) is recommended for all children 2–23 months of age. It also is recommended for certain children 24–59 months of age. Pneumococcal polysaccharide vaccine (PPV) is recommended in addition to PCV for certain high-risk groups (chronic cardiac or pulmonary disease, diabetes mellitus, anatomic asplenia, chronic renal failure, nephrotic syndrome, sickle cell disease, acquired or congenital immunodeficiency).

[g]The second dose of MMR is recommended routinely at age 4–6 years but may be administered during any visit, provided at least 4 weeks have elapsed since receipt of the first dose and that both doses are administered beginning at or after age 12 months. Those who have not previously received the second dose should complete the schedule no later than the routine visit at age 11–12 years.

[h]Varicella vaccine is recommended at any visit on or after age 12 months for susceptible children (ie, those who lack a reliable history of chickenpox and who have not been vaccinated). Susceptible persons aged ≥ 13 years should receive 2 doses given at least 4 weeks apart.

[i]Hepatitis A vaccine is recommended for children and adolescents in selected states and regions and for certain high-risk groups; consult your local public health authority. Children and adolescents in these states, regions, and high-risk groups who have not been immunized against hepatitis A can begin the series during any visit. The 2 doses in the series should be administered ≥ 6 months apart.

[j]Influenza vaccine is recommended annually for children aged ≥ 6 months with certain risk factors [residents of chronic care facilities and patients with chronic cardiopulmonary disorders, metabolic diseases (including diabetes mellitus), hemoglobinopathies, immunosuppression, and renal dysfunction, and household members of persons in groups at high risk]. In addition, healthy children aged 6–23 months are encouraged to receive influenza vaccine if feasible because influenza vaccine in this age group are at substantially increased risk for influenza-related hospitalizations. Children aged ≤ 12 years should receive vaccine dosage appropriate for their age (0.25 mL if aged 6–35 months or 0.5 mL if aged ≥ 3 years). Children aged ≤ 8 years who are receiving influenza vaccine for the first time should receive 2 doses separated by at least 4 weeks.

Source: http://www.cdc.gov/nip

RECOMMENDED ADULT IMMUNIZATION SCHEDULE, UNITED STATES, 2003–2004

by Age Group

Age Group ▶ Vaccine ▼	19–49 Years	50–64 Years	65 Years and Older
Tetanus, diphtheria (Td)*	1 dose booster every 10 years[1]		
Influenza	1 dose annually[2]	1 dose annually[2]	
Pneumococcal (polysaccharide)	1 dose[3,4]	1 dose[3,4]	1 dose[3,4]
Hepatitis B*	3 doses (0, 1–2, 4–6 months)[5]		
Hepatitis A	2 doses (0, 6–12 months)[6]		
Measles, Mumps, Rubella (MMR)*	1 dose if measles, mumps, or rubella vaccination history is unreliable; 2 doses for persons with occupational or other indications[7]		
Varicella*	2 doses (0, 4–8 weeks) for persons who are susceptible[8]		
Meningococcal (polysaccharide)	1 dose[9]		

For all persons in this group   Catch-up on childhood vaccinations   For persons with medical/exposure indications   ■ Contraindicated

*Covered by the Vaccine Injury Compensation Program. For information on how to file a claim, call 800-338-2382. Please also visit www.hrsa.gov/osp/vicp. To file a claim for vaccine injury write: U.S. Court of Federal Claims, 717 Madison Place, N.W., Washington D.C. 20005. 202-219-9657.

This schedule indicates the recommended age groups for routine administration of currently licensed vaccines for persons 19 years of age and older. Licensed combination vaccines may be used whenever any components of the combination are indicated and the vaccine's other components are not contraindicated. Providers should consult the manufacturers' package inserts for detailed recommendations.

Report all clinically significant post-vaccination reactions to the Vaccine Adverse Event Reporting System (VAERS). Reporting forms and instructions on filing a VAERS report are available by calling 800-822-7967 or from the VAERS website at www.vaers.org.

For additional information about the vaccines listed above and contraindications for immunization, visit the National Immunization Program website at www.cdc.gov/nip or call the National Immunization Hotline at 800-232-2522 (English) or 800-232-0233 (Spanish).

Approved by the ACIP, and accepted by the ACOG and the AAFP.

RECOMMENDED ADULT IMMUNIZATION SCHEDULE, UNITED STATES, 2003–2004

by Medical Conditions

Vaccine ▶ ◀ Medical Conditions	Tetanus-diphtheria (Td)*,1	Influenza2	Pneumococcal (polysac-charide)3,4	Hepatitis B*,5	Hepatitis A6	Measles, Mumps, Rubella (MMR)*,7	Varicella*,8
Pregnancy		A					
Diabetes, heart disease, chronic pulmonary disease, chronic liver disease, including chronic alcoholism		B	C		D		
Congenital immunodeficiency, leukemia, lymphoma, generalized malignancy, therapy with alkylating agents, antimetabolites, radiation, or large amounts of corticosteroids			E				F
Renal failure/end stage renal disease, recipients of hemodialysis or clotting factor concentrates			E	G			
Asplenia including elective splenectomy and terminal complement component deficiencies			E, I, J				
HIV infection		H	E, H			L	

Legend:
- For all persons in this group
- Catch-up on childhood vaccinations
- For persons with medical/exposure indications
- ■ Contraindicated

Special Notes for Medical Conditions

A. For women without chronic diseases/conditions, vaccinate if pregnancy will be at 2nd or 3rd trimester during influenza season. For women with chronic diseases/conditions, vaccinate at any time during the pregnancy.

B. Although chronic liver disease and alcoholism are not indicator conditions for influenza vaccination, give 1 dose annually if the patient is ≥ 50 years, has other indicators for influenza vaccine, or if the patient requests vaccination.

C. Asthma is an indicator condition for influenza but not for pneumococcal vaccination.

D. For all persons with chronic liver disease.

E. For persons < 65 years, revaccinate once after 5 years or more have elapsed since initial vaccination.

F. Persons with impaired humoral but not cellular immunity may be vaccinated. MMWR 1999;48 (RR-06):1–5.

G. Hemodialysis patients: use special formulation of vaccine (40 μg/mL) or two 1.0 mL 20 μg doses given at one site. Vaccinate early in the course of renal disease. Assess antibody titers to hep B surface antigen (anti-HBs) levels annually. Administer additional doses if anti-HBs levels decline to < 10 milliinternational units (mIU)/mL.

H. There are no data specifically on risk of severe or complicated influenza infections among persons with asplenia. However, influenza is a risk factor for secondary bacterial infections that may cause severe disease in asplenics.

I. Administer meningococcal vaccine and consider Hib vaccine.

J. Elective splenectomy: vaccinate at least 2 weeks before surgery.

K. Vaccinate as close to diagnosis as possible when CD4 cell counts are highest.

L. Withhold MMR or other measles-containing vaccines from HIV-infected persons with evidence of severe immunosuppression. MMWR 2002;51 (RR-02):22–24.

1. Tetanus and diphtheria (Td)—Adults including pregnant women with uncertain histories of a complete primary vaccination series should receive a primary series of Td. A primary series for adults is 3 doses: the first 2 doses given at least 4 weeks apart and the 3rd dose, 6–12 months after the second. Administer 1 dose if the person had received the primary series and the last vaccination was 10 years ago or longer. Consult MMWR 1991;40 (RR-10):1–21 for administering Td as prophylaxis in wound management. The ACP Task Force on Adult Immunization supports a second opinion for Td use in adults: a single Td booster at age 50 years for persons who have completed the full pediatric series, including the teenage/young adult booster. (*Guide for Adult Immunization,* 3rd ed. ACP 1994:20)

2. Influenza vaccination—Medical indications: chronic disorders of the cardiovascular or pulmonary systems including asthma; chronic metabolic diseases including diabetes mellitus, renal dysfunction, hemoglobinopathies, or immunosuppression [including immunosuppression caused by medications or by human immunodeficiency virus (HIV)]. Occupational indications: health care workers. Other indications: residents of nursing homes and other long-term care facilities; persons likely to transmit influenza to persons at high-risk (in-home caregivers to persons with medical indications, household contacts and out-of-home caregivers of children birth to 23 months of age, or children with asthma or other indicator conditions for influenza vaccination, household members and care givers of elderly and adults with high-risk conditions); and anyone who wishes to be vaccinated. For healthy persons aged 5–49 years without high risk conditions, either the inactivated vaccine or the intranasally administered influenza vaccine (Flumist) may be given. [MMWR 2003;52 (RR-8):1–36; MMWR 2003;52 (RR-13);12]

3. Pneumococcal polysaccharide vaccination—Medical indications: chronic disorders of the pulmonary system (excluding asthma), cardiovascular diseases, diabetes mellitus, chronic liver diseases including liver disease as a result of alcohol abuse (eg, cirrhosis), chronic renal failure or nephrotic syndrome, functional or anatomic asplenia (eg, sickle cell disease or splenectomy), immunosuppressive conditions (eg, congenital immunodeficiency, HIV infection, leukemia, lymphoma, multiple myeloma, Hodgkin's disease, generalized malignancy, organ or bone marrow transplantation), chemotherapy with alkylating agents, anti-metabolites, or long-term systemic corticosteroids. Geographic/other indications: Alaskan Natives and certain American Indian populations. Other indications: residents of nursing homes and other long-term care facilities. [MMWR 1997;47 (RR-8):1–24] Revaccination with pneumococcal polysaccharide vaccine—One-time revaccination after 5 years for persons with chronic renal failure or nephrotic syndrome, functional or anatomic asplenia (eg, sickle cell disease or splenectomy), immunosuppressive conditions (eg, congenital immunodeficiency, HIV infection, leukemia, lymphoma, multiple myeloma, Hodgkin's disease, generalized malignancy, organ or bone marrow transplantation), chemotherapy with alkylating agents, anti-metabolites, or long-term systemic corticosteroids. For persons 65 and older, one-time revaccination if they were vaccinated 5 or more years previously and were aged less than 65 years at the time of primary vaccination. [MMWR 1997;47 (RR-8):1–24]

5. Hepatitis B vaccination—Medical indications: hemodialysis patients, patients who receive clotting-factor concentrates. Occupational indications: health care workers and public-safety workers who have exposure to blood in the workplace, persons in training in schools of medicine, dentistry, nursing, laboratory technology, and other allied health professions. Behavioral indications: injecting drug users, persons with more than one sex partner in the previous 6 months, persons with a recently acquired sexually transmitted disease (STD), all clients in STD clinics, men who have sex with men. Other indications: household contacts and sex partners of persons with chronic HBV infection, clients and staff of institutions for the developmentally disabled, international travelers who will be in countries with high or intermediate prevalence of chronic HBV infection for more than 6 months, inmates of correctional facilities. [MMWR 1991;40 (RR-13): 1–25; www.cdc.gov/travel/diseases/hbv.htm]

6. Hepatitis A vaccination—For the combined HepA-HepB vaccine use 3 doses at 0, 1, 6 months. Medical indications: persons with clotting-factor disorders or chronic liver disease. Behavioral indications: men who have sex with men, users of injecting and noninjecting illegal drugs. Occupational indications: persons working with HAV-infected primates or with HAV in a research laboratory setting. Other indications: persons traveling to or working in countries that have high or intermediate endemicity of hepatitis A. [MMWR 1999;48 (RR-12):1–37; www.cdc.gov/travel/diseases/hav.htm]

7. Measles, Mumps, Rubella vaccination (MMR)—Measles component: Adults born before 1957 may be considered immune to measles. Adults born in or after 1957 should receive at least one dose of MMR unless they have a medical contraindication, documentation of at least one dose or other acceptable evidence of immunity. A second dose of MMR is recommended for adults who:

- are recently exposed to measles or in an outbreak setting
- were previously vaccinated with killed measles vaccine
- were vaccinated with an unknown vaccine between 1963 and 1967
- are students in postsecondary educational institutions
- work in health care facilities
- plan to travel internationally

Mumps component: 1 dose of MMR should be adequate for protection. Rubella component: Give 1 dose of MMR to women whose rubella vaccination history is unreliable and counsel women to avoid becoming pregnant for 4 weeks after vaccination. For women of child-bearing age, regardless of birth year, routinely determine rubella immunity and counsel women regarding congenital rubella syndrome. Do not vaccinate pregnant women or those planning to become pregnant in the next 4 weeks. If pregnant and susceptible, vaccinate as early in postpartum period as possible. [MMWR 1998;47 (RR-8):1–57; MMWR 2001;50:1117]

8. Varicella vaccination—Recommended for all persons who do not have reliable clinical history of varicella infection, or serological evidence of varicella zoster virus (VZV) infection who may be at high risk for exposure or transmission. This includes health care workers and family contacts of immunosuppressed patients, those who live or work in environments where transmission is likely (eg, teachers of young children, day care employees, and residents and staff members in institutional settings), persons who live or work in environments where VZV transmission can occur (eg, college students, inmates and staff members of correctional institutions, and military personnel), adolescents and adults living in households with children, women who are not pregnant but who may become pregnant in the future, international travelers who are not immune to infection. Note: Greater than 95% of U.S. born adults are immune to VZV. Do not vaccinate pregnant women or those planning to become pregnant in the next 4 weeks. If pregnant and susceptible, vaccinate as early in the postpartum period as possible. [MMWR 1996;45 (RR-11):1–36; MMWR 1999;48 (RR-6):1–5]

9. Meningococcal vaccine (quadrivalent polysaccharide for serogroups A, C, Y, and W-135)—Consider vaccination for persons with medical indications: adults with terminal complement component deficiencies, with anatomic or functional asplenia. Other indications: travelers to countries in which disease is hyperendemic or epidemic ("meningitis belt" of sub-Saharan Africa, Mecca, Saudi Arabia for Haij). Revaccination at 3–5 years may be indicated for persons at high risk for infection (eg, persons residing in areas in which disease is epidemic). Counsel college freshmen, especially those who live in dormitories, regarding meningococcal disease and the vaccine so that they can make an educated decision about receiving the vaccination. [MMWR 2000;49: (RR-7): 1–20] Note: The AAFP recommends that colleges should take the lead on providing education on meningococcal infection and vaccination and offer it to those who are interested. Physicians need not initiate discussion of the meningococcal quadrivalent polysaccharide vaccine as part of routine medical care.

Recommendations for using smallpox vaccine in a pre-event vaccination program:

Smallpox vaccination is recommended for persons designated by public health authorities to conduct investigations and follow-up of initial smallpox cases that might necessitate direct patient contact. ACIP recommends that each state and territory establish and maintain ≥ 1 smallpox response team. Pre-event vaccination is contraindicated for persons with a history or presence of eczema or atopic dermatitis; who have other acute, chronic, or exfoliative skin conditions; who have conditions associated with immunosuppression; who are aged < 1 year; who have a serious allergy to any component of the vaccine; or who are pregnant or breast-feeding, and their household contacts. ACIP does note recommend pre-event vaccination for children and adolescents aged < 18 years. [MMWR 2003;52 (RR-7): 1–16]

Source: www.cdc.gov/nip

3
Disease Management

ADULT PATIENT WITH ALLERGIC RHINITIS: DIAGNOSIS AND MANAGEMENT
Source: American Academy of Allergy, Asthma and Immunology (AAAAI) and
American College of Allergy, Asthma and Immunology (ACAAI)

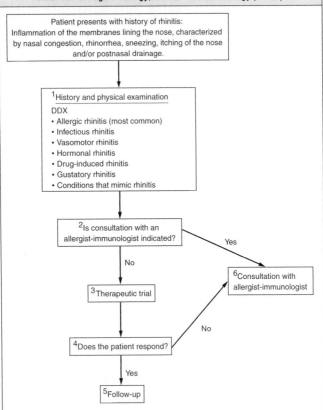

Patient presents with history of rhinitis:
Inflammation of the membranes lining the nose, characterized
by nasal congestion, rhinorrhea, sneezing, itching of the nose
and/or postnasal drainage.

[1] History and physical examination

DDX
- Allergic rhinitis (most common)
- Infectious rhinitis
- Vasomotor rhinitis
- Hormonal rhinitis
- Drug-induced rhinitis
- Gustatory rhinitis
- Conditions that mimic rhinitis

[2] Is consultation with an allergist-immunologist indicated?

Yes

No

[6] Consultation with allergist-immunologist

[3] Therapeutic trial

No

[4] Does the patient respond?

Yes

[5] Follow-up

Source: Adapted from Diagnosis and Management of Rhinitis: Parameter Documents
of the Joint Task Force on Practice Parameters in Allergy, Asthma and Immunology.
American Academy of Allergy, Asthma and Immunology (AAAAI) and American College
of Allergy, Asthma and Immunology (ACAAI). 1998. (http://www.jcaai.org)

Adult Rhinitis Algorithm: Notes

1. History: (a) presenting symptoms (eg, rhinorrhea, nasal congestion, sneezing, ocular sx); (b) length of symptomatology; (c) past medications taken for rhinitis, their effectiveness and adverse effects; (d) other medications; (e) degree to which rhinitis sx interfere with patient's ability to function and affect patient's quality of life; (f) seasonality and known triggers; (g) other medical conditions; (h) complications (eg, otitis media); (i) associated comorbid conditions (eg, asthma). Physical exam: (a) evaluation of nose—appearance of nasal mucous membranes, patency of nasal passageways, quality and quantity of nasal discharge; (b) evaluation of ears, eyes, throat, and lungs.

2. Consider initial referral if: (a) need to define allergic/environmental triggers of rhinitis sx; (b) need for more intense education; (c) requires multiple medications over a prolonged period of time.

3. (a) **Avoidance of inciting factors.**

   (b) **Oral antihistamines:** Effective in reducing symptoms of itching, sneezing, and rhinorrhea. First line therapy for treatment of allergic rhinitis. Little objective effect on nasal congestion. Second generation antihistamines that are associated with less risk or no risk for sedation and performance impairment should usually be considered before sedating antihistamines.

   (c) **Intranasal antihistamines:** Appropriate first line treatment. May help reduce nasal congestion. Sedation may occur from systemic absorption.

   (d) **Oral decongestants:** Can effectively reduce nasal congestion. Can cause insomnia, anorexia, excessive nervousness. May increase BP.

   (e) **Nasally inhaled steroids:** Most effective medication class for controlling sx of allergic rhinitis. May be considered for initial tx without a prior trial of antihistamines and/or oral decongestants, and should be considered before initiating tx with systemic corticosteroids.

   (f) **Oral corticosteroids:** Should be reserved for severe cases of rhinitis. Short burst (5–7 days) preferred over depot parenteral corticosteroids, which should be avoided.

   (g) **Intranasal cromolyn sodium:** Can reduce sx of allergic rhinitis in some patients; is most likely effective if initiated before sx become severe.

   (h) **Intranasal anticholinergics:** May effectively reduce rhinorrhea but have no effect on other nasal sx.

4. Reasons for referral: (a) duration of rhinitis sx > 3 months; (b) complications of rhinitis (eg, otitis media, sinusitis, nasal polyps); (c) comorbid conditions (eg, asthma); (d) requires oral corticosteroids for rhinitis; (e) symptoms interfere with patient's ability to function; (f) symptoms significantly decrease patient's quality of life; (g) treatment with medications for rhinitis are ineffective or produce adverse events; (h) need to define allergic/environmental triggers of rhinitis sx; (i) need for more intense education; (j) requires multiple medications over a prolonged period of time.

5. If initial tx successful, follow patient to assure continued control of sx, maintenance of improved quality of life, absence of medication side effects, and reinforce education.

6. Additional examination may include: rhinoscopy, immediate hypersensitivity skin tests, or in vitro tests to confirm an underlying allergic basis for symptoms. Neither total serum IgE nor total circulating eosinophil counts are routinely indicated as they are neither sensitive nor specific for allergic rhinitis. Specific tests may be necessary for co-existing conditions (eg, asthma, nasal polyps, sinusitis). Specific immunotherapy may be beneficial.

Source: American Academy of Otolaryngic Allergy (AAOA). Allergic rhinitis: clinical practice guideline. Otolaryngol Head Neck Surg 1996;115(1):115–122.

PHARMACOLOGICAL MANAGEMENT OF ARTHRITIS OF HIP AND KNEE
Source: American College of Rheumatology, AAOS

Step-1 | **Non-Pharmacologic Therapy**

- Patient education
- Self-management programs
- Personalized social support through telephone contact
- Weight loss (if overweight)
- Aerobic exercise programs
- Physical therapy
  - Range-of-motion
  - Muscle-strengthening[1]

- Assistive devices for ambulation
- Patellar taping
- Appropriate footwear
- Lateral-wedged insoles (for genu varum)
- Occupational therapy
  - Joint protection
  - Activities of daily living

⇩ *inadequate symptom relief*

Step-2 | **Acetaminophen[2]** (total daily dose not to exceed 4.0 gm/day)
*If moderate-to-severe **inflammation present**, consider **NSAID first**.[3]*

⇩ *inadequate symptom relief*

Step-3 | **Evaluate Renal and Gastrointestinal Risk**

Renal Risk Present?
creatinine ≥ 2.0 mg/dL
+
(1 of the following)
age ≥ 65 yrs, hypertension, congestive heart failure, OR diuretic or ACE inhibitor therapy

Yes →

No ↓

GI Risk Present?
(at least 1 of the following)
age ≥ 65 yrs
comorbidity
oral glucocorticoid Rx
peptic ulcer disease Hx
upper GI bleed Hx
anticoagulant Rx

Yes →

No ↓

Treatment Options

Non-NSAID Oral Therapy
- Tramadol
- Salsalate

Intraarticular therapy
- Glucocorticoids
- Hyaluronan[4]
Topical therapy[5]
- Capsaicin
- Methylsalicylate

Oral Therapy
- Salsalate
- COX-2 inhibitors[6]
- NSAID + misoprostol or proton pump inhibitor
- Tramadol

Oral Therapy
- Non-selective NSAID, or other therapies above[7]

⇩ *inadequate symptom relief*

Step-4 | **Consider additional or alternative therapies**
- Opioid therapy
- Total joint arthroplasty[8]

Source: Adapted from American College of Rheumatology Subcommittee on Osteoarthritis Guidelines. Recommendations for the Medical Management of Osteoarthritis of the Hip and Knee. Arthritis and Rheumatism 2000;43:1905–1915.

Similar management algorithm offered by AAOS—adds recommendations for radiographs and for knee aspiration (www.aaos.org).

FOOTNOTES

1. Quadriceps weakness may precede, initiate, and exacerbate knee osteoarthritis. (Rheum Dis Clin North Am 1999;25:283–398)

2. For many patients with mild-moderate osteoarthritis, pain relief with acetaminophen is comparable to NSAID. (Semin Arthritis Rheum 1997;27:755–770)

3. NSAIDs appear to be superior to acetaminophen in patients with severe pain related to osteoarthritis. (Arthritis Rheum 2000;43:378–385, J Rheumatol 2000;27:1020–1027)

4. Hyaluronan intraarticular therapy has only been evaluated in knee osteoarthritis.

5. Topical therapy primarily indicated for mild-to-moderate pain related to osteoarthritis of the knee. There are no studies of topical therapy for hip osteoarthritis.

6. COX-2 inhibitors (celecoxib and rofecoxib) are as efficacious as non-selective NSAIDs, but not more efficacious. In contrast to non-selective NSAIDs, COX-2 inhibitors do not impair platelet function or bleeding time.

7. Use of concomitant gastroprotective therapy with misoprostol or a proton pump inhibitor is not recommended in the low-risk patient.

8. In a randomized trial, 180 patients with osteoarthritis of the knee were randomly assigned to receive arthroscopic debridement, arthroscopic lavage, or placebo surgery. The outcomes (pain, physical function) after arthroscopic debridement or lavage were no better than those after the placebo procedure over 24 months of follow-up. (NEJM 2002;347:81–88) However, total joint arthroplasty provides marked pain relief and functional improvement in the vast majority of patients with osteoarthritis, and has been shown to be cost-effective in selected patients. An NIH Consensus conference recommends total hip replacement when "radiographic evidence of joint damage and moderate-to-severe persistent pain and disability, or both, that is not substantially relieved by an extended course of non-surgical management" is present.

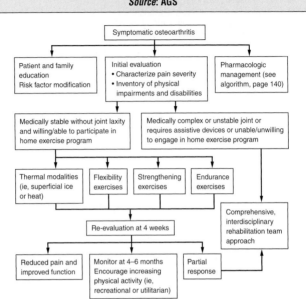

**EXERCISE PRESCRIPTION FOR OLDER ADULTS
WITH OSTEOARTHRITIS PAIN**
Source: AGS

Symptomatic osteoarthritis

- Patient and family education
  Risk factor modification
- Initial evaluation
  • Characterize pain severity
  • Inventory of physical impairments and disabilities
- Pharmacologic management (see algorithm, page 140)

Medically stable without joint laxity and willing/able to participate in home exercise program

Medically complex or unstable joint or requires assistive devices or unable/unwilling to engage in home exercise program

- Thermal modalities (ie, superficial ice or heat)
- Flexibility exercises
- Strengthening exercises
- Endurance exercises

Comprehensive, interdisciplinary rehabilitation team approach

Re-evaluation at 4 weeks

- Reduced pain and improved function
- Monitor at 4–6 months Encourage increasing physical activity (ie, recreational or utilitarian)
- Partial response

Major risk factors for osteoarthritis: obesity, muscle weakness, heavy physical activity, inactivity, trauma, reduced proprioception, poor joint biomechanics, age, female gender, inheritance, congenital (ie, malformations). Adapted from American Geriatrics Society Consensus Practice Recommendations. (JAGS 2001;49:808–823)

STEPWISE APPROACH FOR MANAGING ASTHMA IN ADULTS AND CHILDREN OLDER THAN 5 YEARS OF AGE

ASTHMA: SEVERITY CLASSIFICATION
Source: NHLBI

GOALS OF ASTHMA TREATMENT

	Clinical Features before Treatment[a]		
	Symptoms[b]	Nighttime Symptoms	Lung Function
STEP 4 Severe Persistent	Continual symptoms Limited physical activity Frequent exacerbations	Frequent	FEV1 or PEF < 60% predicted PEF variability > 30%
STEP 3 Moderate Persistent	Daily symptoms Daily use of inhaled short-acting beta$_2$-agonist Exacerbations affect activity Exacerbations = 2 times a week; may last days	> 1 time a week	FEV1 or PEF > 60% – < 80% predicted PEF variability > 30%
STEP 2 Mild Persistent	Symptoms > 2 times a week but < 1 time a day Exacerbations may affect activity	> 2 times a month	FEV1 or PEF = 80% predicted PEF variability 20%–30%
STEP 1 Mild Intermittent	Symptoms ≤ 2 times a week Asymptomatic and normal PEF between exacerbations Exacerbations brief (from a few hours to a few days); intensity may vary	≤ 2 times a month	FEV1 or PEF = 80% predicted PEF variability < 20%

ASTHMA: SEVERITY CLASSIFICATION
Source: NHLBI

[a]The presence of one of the features of severity is sufficient to place a patient in that category. An individual should be assigned to the most severe grade in which any feature occurs. The characteristics noted in this table are general and may overlap because asthma is highly variable. Furthermore, an individual's classification may change over time.

[b]Patients at any level of severity can have mild, moderate, or severe exacerbations. Some patients with intermittent asthma experience severe and life-threatening exacerbations separated by long periods of normal lung function and no symptoms.

Source: National Heart, Lung and Blood Institute; NIH. http://www.nhlbi.nih.gov/guidelines/asthma/index.htm

ASTHMA: TREATMENT
Source: NHLBI

STEPWISE APPROACH FOR MANAGING ASTHMA IN ADULTS AND CHILDREN OLDER THAN 5 YEARS OF AGE: TREATMENT			
	Long-Term Control	**Quick Relief**	**Education**
STEP 4 Severe Persistent	Daily medications: Anti-inflammatory: inhaled corticosteroid (high dose) AND Long-acting bronchodilator: either long-acting inhaled beta$_2$-agonist, sustained-release theophylline, or long-acting beta$_2$-agonist tablets AND Corticosteroid tablets or syrup long term (make repeat attempts to reduce systemic steroids and maintain control with high-dose inhaled steroids)	Short-acting bronchodilator: inhaled beta$_2$-agonists as needed for symptoms Intensity of treatment will depend on severity of exacerbation. Use of short-acting inhaled beta$_2$-agonists on a daily basis, or increasing use, indicates the need for additional long-term control therapy.	Steps 2 and 3 actions plus: Refer to individual education/counseling.

ASTHMA: TREATMENT *Source:* **NHLBI**		

STEPWISE APPROACH FOR MANAGING ASTHMA IN ADULTS AND CHILDREN OLDER THAN 5 YEARS OF AGE: TREATMENT (CONTINUED)

	Long-Term Control	Quick Relief	Education
STEP 3 **Moderate** **Persistent**	Daily medication: Either Anti-inflammatory: inhaled corticosteroid (medium dose) OR Inhaled corticosteroid (low-medium dose) and add a long-acting bronchodilator, especially for nighttime symptoms; either long-acting inhaled beta₂-agonist, sustained-release theophylline, or long-acting beta₂-agonist tablets If needed: Anti-inflammatory: inhaled corticosteroids (medium-high dose) AND Long-acting bronchodilator, especially for nighttime symptoms: either long-acting inhaled beta₂-agonist, sustained-release theophylline, or long-acting beta₂-agonist tablets	Short-acting bronchodilator: inhaled beta₂-agonists as needed for symptoms. Intensity of treatment will depend on severity of exacerbation. Use of short-acting inhaled beta₂-agonists on a daily basis, or increasing use, indicates the need for additional long-term control therapy.	Step 1 actions plus: Teach self-monitoring. Refer to group education if available. Review and update self-management plan.

ASTHMA: TREATMENT Source: NHLBI			
STEPWISE APPROACH FOR MANAGING ASTHMA IN ADULTS AND CHILDREN OLDER THAN 5 YEARS OF AGE: TREATMENT (CONTINUED)			
	Long-Term Control	Quick Relief	Education
STEP 2 Mild Persistent	One daily medication: Anti-inflammatory: either inhaled corticosteroid (low doses) or cromolyn or nedocromil (children usually begin with a trial of cromolyn or nedocromil). Sustained-release theophylline to serum concentration of 5–15 mg/L is an alternative, but not preferred, therapy. Zafirlukast or zileuton may also be considered for patients > 12 years of age, although their position in therapy is not fully established.	Short-acting bronchodilator: inhaled beta$_2$-agonists as needed for symptoms. Intensity of treatment will depend on severity of exacerbation. Use of short-acting inhaled beta$_2$-agonists on a daily basis, or increasing use, indicates the need for additional long-term control therapy.	Step 1 actions plus: Teach self-monitoring. Refer to group education if available. Review and update self-management plan.

ASTHMA: TREATMENT		
Source: NHLBI		

STEPWISE APPROACH FOR MANAGING ASTHMA IN ADULTS AND CHILDREN OLDER THAN 5 YEARS OF AGE: TREATMENT (CONTINUED)

	Long-Term Control	Quick Relief	Education
STEP 1 Mild Intermittent	No daily medication needed	Short-acting bronchodilator: inhaled beta$_2$-agonists as needed for symptoms. Intensity of treatment will depend on severity of exacerbation. Use of short-acting inhaled beta$_2$-agonists more than 2 times a week may indicate the need to initiate long-term control therapy.	Teach basic facts about asthma. Teach inhaler/spacer/holding chamber technique. Discuss roles of medications. Develop self-management plan. Develop action plan for when and how to take rescue actions, especially for patients with a history of severe exacerbations. Discuss appropriate environmental control measures to avoid exposure to known allergens and irritants.

ASTHMA: TREATMENT
Source: NHLBI

STEPWISE APPROACH FOR MANAGING ASTHMA IN ADULTS AND CHILDREN OLDER THAN 5 YEARS OF AGE: TREATMENT (CONTINUED)

Step down: Review treatment every 16 months; a gradual stepwise reduction in treatment may be possible.	Step up: If control is not maintained, consider step up. First, review patient medication technique, adherence, and environmental control (avoidance of allergens or other factors that contribute to asthma severity).

Note: The stepwise approach presents general guidelines to assist clinical decision making; it is not intended to be a specific prescription. Asthma is highly variable; clinicians should tailor specific medication plans to the needs and circumstances of individual patients.

Gain control as quickly as possible; then decrease treatment to the least medication necessary to maintain control. Gaining control may be accomplished by either starting treatment at the step most appropriate to the initial severity of the condition or starting at a higher level or therapy (eg, a course of systemic corticosteroids or higher dose of inhaled corticosteroids).

A rescue course of systemic corticosteroids may be needed at any time and at any step.

Some patients with intermittent asthma experience severe and life-threatening exacerbations separated by long periods of normal lung function and no symptoms. This may be especially common with exacerbations provoked by respiratory infections. A short course of systemic corticosteroids is recommended.

At each step, patients should control their environment to avoid or control factors that make their asthma worse (eg, allergens, irritants); this requires specific diagnosis and education.

Referral to an asthma specialist for consultation or co-management is recommended if there are difficulties achieving or maintaining control of asthma or if the patient requires step 4 care. Referral may be considered if the patient requires step 3 care.

Source: NHLBI; NIH. http://www.nhlbi.nih.gov/guidelines/asthma/index.htm

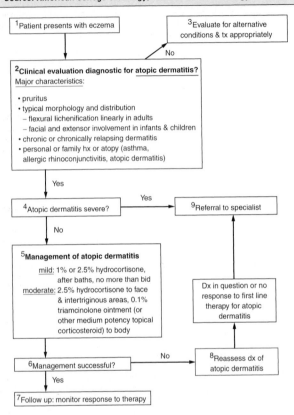

ATOPIC DERMATITIS: EVALUATION & MANAGEMENT ALGORITHM
Source: **American College of Allergy, Asthma and Immunology and AAD**

[1] Patient presents with eczema

[3] Evaluate for alternative conditions & tx appropriately

No

[2] **Clinical evaluation diagnostic for atopic dermatitis?**
Major characteristics:

- pruritus
- typical morphology and distribution
  - flexural lichenification linearly in adults
  - facial and extensor involvement in infants & children
- chronic or chronically relapsing dermatitis
- personal or family hx or atopy (asthma, allergic rhinoconjunctivitis, atopic dermatitis)

Yes

[4] Atopic dermatitis severe?

Yes

[9] Referral to specialist

No

[5] **Management of atopic dermatitis**

mild: 1% or 2.5% hydrocortisone, after baths, no more than bid
moderate: 2.5% hydrocortisone to face & intertriginous areas, 0.1% triamcinolone ointment (or other medium potency topical corticosteroid) to body

Dx in question or no response to first line therapy for atopic dermatitis

[6] Management successful?

No

[8] Reassess dx of atopic dermatitis

Yes

[7] Follow up: monitor response to therapy

Source: Adapted from Disease Management of Atopic Dermatitis: A Practice Parameter. Am Allergy Asthma Immunol 1997 Sep; 79(3):197–211. (http://www.jcaai.org) and Guidelines of Care for Atopic Dermatitis, AAD, 2003 (www.aad.org).

Atopic Dermatitis: Evaluation and Management Algorithm Notes

1. **Eczema** refers to a pruritic dermatitis that includes a long list of differential diagnoses (see notes 2 and 3).

2. **Other characteristics of atopic dermatitis** (in the absence of an atopic history, 3 or more required for diagnosis): xerosis; ichthyosis/palmar hyperlinearity/keratosis pilaris; immediate, Type I skin test response; hand and/or foot dermatitis; cheilitis; nipple eczema; susceptibility to cutaneous infections; erythroderma; early age of onset; impaired cell-mediated immunity; recurrent conjunctivitis; infraorbital fold; keratoconus; anterior subscapular cataracts; elevated total serum immunoglobulin E; peripheral blood eosinophils. **History:** pruritic nature of rash, age of onset, duration, triggers, seasonal variation, eye complications, environmental exposures, chronicity, distribution of rash. **Physical examination:** morphology and distribution of the atopic skin lesions, especially noting diffuse xerosis, erythema, excoriation, papulation, crusting/oozing/ pustules indicative of infection, scaling, lichenification. Look for associated characteristics. **Laboratory testing:** skin or in vitro testing for specific allergens. The majority of patients have elevated serum IgE and eosinophilia; these findings are not useful in guiding clinical decisions. A diagnosis of atopic dermatitis cannot be made solely on the basis of laboratory testing.

3. **Differential diagnosis of atopic dermatitis**
   - Immunodeficiencies: Wiskott-Aldrich syndrome, DiGeorge syndrome, Hyper-IgE syndrome, severe combined immune deficiency
   - Metabolic diseases: Phenylketonuria, tyrosinemia, histidinemia, multiple carboxylase deficiency, essential fatty acid deficiency
   - Neoplastic disease: Cutaneous T-cell lymphoma, histiocytosis X, Sézary syndrome
   - Infection and infestation: Candida, herpes simplex, *Staphylococcus aureus*, *Sarcoptes scabiei*
   - Dermatitis: Contact, seborrheic, psoriasis

4. **Severe atopic dermatitis:**
   - More than 20% skin involvement (or 10% skin involvement if affected areas include the eyelids, hands, or intertriginous areas)
   - Extensive skin involvement and erythrodermic, at risk for exfoliation
   - Requiring ongoing or frequent treatment with high potency topical glucocorticoids or systemic glucocorticoids
   - Requiring hospitalization for severe eczema or skin infections related to atopic dermatitis
   - Ocular or infectious complications
   - Significant disruption of quality of life

5. Treatment of atopic dermatitis is directed at symptom relief and reduction of cutaneous inflammation. Characterization of each patient's atopic dermatitis severity and reduction of exacerbating factors are critical for effective management. All patients require skin hydration in combination with an effective emollient. Potential trigger factors should be identified and eliminated. Calcineurin inhibitors, pimecrolimus, and tacrolimus have been shown to reduce the extent, severity, and symptoms of atopic dermatitis. Tar may be associated with therapeutic benefits, but is limited by compliance. Short-term adjunctive use of topical doxepin may aid in the reduction of pruritus, but side effects may limit usefulness. Patients with atopic dermatitis are commonly colonized with *Staphylococcus aureus*. Without signs of infection, oral antibiotics have minimal therapeutic effect on the dermatitis. Oral antibiotics can be highly beneficial when skin infection is present. Topical antibiotics can be effective when infection is present; development of resistance is a concern.

6. Response to therapy is classified as complete response, partial response, or treatment failure. Because atopic dermatitis is a chronic relapsing skin condition, most patients will have a partial response with reduction in pruritus and extent of skin disease.

7. Follow-up is required to monitor the patient's response to therapy and adjust medications and skin care according to severity of illness. A plan should be established to step up medications for flare-ups and to step down medications when the illness is under control.

8. In any patient who fails to respond to treatment, it is important to reassess the diagnosis to be certain the patient has atopic dermatitis. In patients presenting after the age of 16 years, consider contact dermatitis. In patients presenting as adults, consider cutaneous T-cell lymphoma.

9. The patient who does not respond to first-line therapy, or who has severe atopic dermatitis (note 4) is highly challenging and requires a multidisciplinary approach that may exceed the resources of the primary care physician. For these patients, consultation with a specialist who is skilled in the management of patients with severe atopic dermatitis can be beneficial.

ATRIAL FIBRILLATION: EVALUATION & MANAGEMENT

Source: American Heart Association/American College of Cardiology/European Society of Cardiology

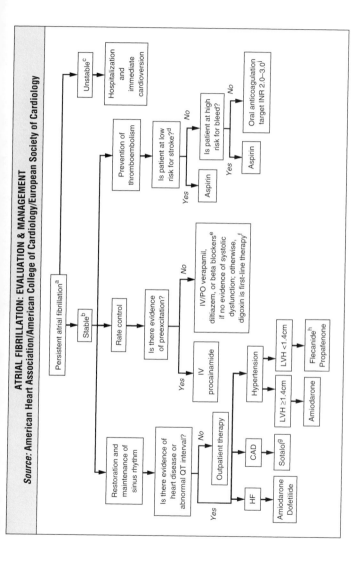

ATRIAL FIBRILLATION: EVALUATION & MANAGEMENT (CONTINUED)
Source: AHA/ACC/European Society of Cardiology

[a] Paroxysmal atrial fibrillation episodes last more than 30 seconds, but ≤ 7 days. If ≥ 2 episodes, designate "persistent."

[b] If minimal or no symptoms, anticoagulation, and rate control, "as needed."

[c] Evidence of Wolff-Parkinson-White syndrome of preexcitation, hypotension, or congestive heart failure; ECG evidence of acute MI or symptomatic hypotension, angina, or heart failure.

[d] Patients at high stroke risk (thromboembolic rates > 5/year) include those with a history of hypertension, prior stroke/transient ischemic attack, diabetes, age > 65 years, impaired systolic function, and enlarged left atrial size. Low-risk patients have a thromboembolic risk of 1%–1.5% per year. (Arch Intern Med 1994;154:1449; Am Intern Med 1992;116:1).

[e] Beta-blockers are especially effective in the setting of thyrotoxicosis or increased sympathetic tone (eg, alcohol withdrawal).

[f] If rate is difficult to control with pharmacologic therapy, consider AV node ablation or modification.

[g] Second-line therapy: amiodalarone, dofetilide; third-line: disopyramide, procainamide, quinidine.

[h] Second-line therapy: amiodalarone, dofetilide, sotalol; third-line: disopyramide, procainamide, quinidine.

[i] Consider range 1.6 to 2.5 in patients age > 75 years with increased risk of bleeding complications.

CAD, coronary artery disease; HF, heart failure; LVH, left ventricular hypertrophy.

Source: Adapted from AHA subcommittee on Electrocardiography and Electrophysiology. Circulation 1996;93:1262; and ACC/AHA/ESC, J Am Coll Card 2001;38:1265.

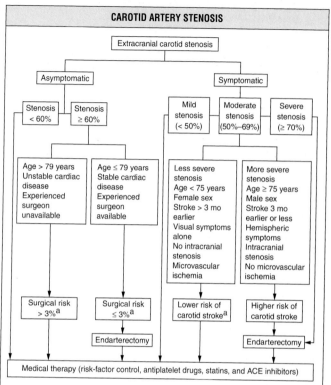

CAROTID ARTERY STENOSIS

Extracranial carotid stenosis

Asymptomatic

- Stenosis < 60%
- Stenosis ≥ 60%

Age > 79 years / Unstable cardiac disease / Experienced surgeon unavailable

Age ≤ 79 years / Stable cardiac disease / Experienced surgeon available

Surgical risk > 3%[a]

Surgical risk ≤ 3%[a] → Endarterectomy

Symptomatic

- Mild stenosis (< 50%)
- Moderate stenosis (50%–69%)
- Severe stenosis (≥ 70%)

Less severe stenosis / Age < 75 years / Female sex / Stroke > 3 mo earlier / Visual symptoms alone / No intracranial stenosis / Microvascular ischemia

More severe stenosis / Age ≥ 75 years / Male sex / Stroke 3 mo earlier or less / Hemispheric symptoms / Intracranial stenosis / No microvascular ischemia

Lower risk of carotid stroke[a]

Higher risk of carotid stroke → Endarterectomy

Medical therapy (risk-factor control, antiplatelet drugs, statins, and ACE inhibitors)

Source: Adapted from The Guidelines of the American Heart Association and the National Stroke Association. Other factors not included in the figure may also be relevant in risk stratification (eg, the results of cardiac evaluation or hemodynamic testing). Sacco RL. NEJM 2001;345;113.

[a]Retrospective review of 1370 CEA (1990–1999) at 1 teaching hospital: no significant difference in incidence of perioperative stroke or death in those with ≥ 1 vs. no risk factors. 30-day mortality significantly greater (2.8% vs. 0.3%, $p = 0.04$) in those with ≥ 2 vs. no risk factors. (J Vasc Surg 2003;37:1191–1199)

CATARACT IN ADULTS: EVALUATION & MANAGEMENT ALGORITHM
Source: AHRQ

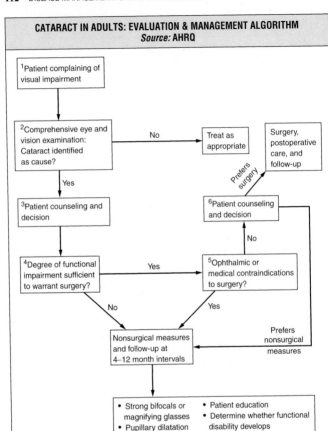

Sources: Adapted from Cataract in Adults: Management of Functional Impairment (Clinical Practice Guideline). Publication No. AHCPR 93-0542. Rockville, MD: Agency for Health Care Research and Quality Public Health Service, U.S. Department of Health and Human Services, February 1993.

American Academy of Ophthalmology and American Society of Cataract and Refractive Surgery. White Paper on Cataract Surgery, 1996.

American Optometric Association Consensus Panel on Care of the Adult Patient with Cataract. Optometric Clinical Practice Guideline: Care of the Adult Patient with Cataract. Updated 3/30/99.

Cataract in Adults: Evaluation & Management Algorithm Notes

1. Cataract evaluation and management should begin only when patients complain of a visual problem or impairment. Identifying impairment in visual function during routine history and physical examination constitutes sound medical practice.

2. Essential elements of the comprehensive eye and vision examination:
   - Patient history. Consider cataracts if: acute or gradual onset of vision loss; vision problems under special conditions (eg, low contrast, glare); difficulties performing various visual tasks. Ask about: refractive history; previous ocular disease; amblyopia; eye surgery; trauma; general health history; medications; and allergies. In addition, it is critical to describe the actual impact of the cataract on the person's function and quality of life. There are several instruments available for assessing functional impairment related to cataract, including VF-14, Activities of Daily Vision Scale, and Visual Activities Questionnaire.
   - Ocular examination, including: Snellen acuity and refraction; measurement of intraocular pressure; assessment of pupillary function; external examination; slit-lamp examination; and dilated examination of fundus.
   - Supplemental testing: May be necessary to assess and document the extent of the functional disability and to determine whether other diseases may limit preoperative or postoperative vision.

   Most elderly patients presenting with visual problems do not have a cataract that causes functional impairment. Refractive error, macular degeneration, and glaucoma are common alternative etiologies for visual impairment.

3. Once cataract has been identified as the cause of visual disability, patients should be counseled concerning the nature of the problem, its natural history, and the existence of both surgical and nonsurgical approaches to management. The principal factor that should guide decision making with regard to surgery is the extent to which the cataract impairs the ability to function in daily life. The findings of the physical examination should corroborate that the cataract is the major contributing cause of the functional impairment, and that there is a reasonable expectation that managing the cataract will positively impact the patient's functional activity. Visual acuity is not the *sole* determining factor and should not be used as a threshold value.

4. Patients who complain of mild to moderate limitation in activities due to a visual problem, those whose corrected acuities are near 20/40, and those who do not yet wish to undergo surgery may be offered nonsurgical measures for improving visual function. Indications for surgery: cataract-impaired vision no longer meets the patient's needs; evidence of lens-induced disease (eg, phakomorphic glaucoma, phakolytic glaucoma); necessary to visualize the fundus in an eye that has the potential for sight (eg, diabetic patient who is at risk of diabetic nephropathy).

5. Contraindications to surgery: the patient does not desire surgery; glasses or visual aids provide satisfactory functional vision; surgery will not improve visual function; the patient's quality of life is not compromised; the patient is unable to undergo surgery because of coexisting medical or ocular conditions; a legal consent cannot be obtained; or the patient is unable to obtain adequate postoperative care. Routine preoperative medical testing (12-lead EKG, CBC, measurement of serum electrolytes, BUN, creatinine, and glucose), while commonly performed in patients scheduled to undergo cataract surgery, does not appear to measurably increase the safety of the surgery.

6. Patients with significant functional and visual impairment due to cataract who have no contraindications to surgery should be counseled regarding the expected risks and benefits of surgery and alternatives to surgery.

EVALUATING THE ADULT WITH ACUTE, NON-TRAUMATIC CHEST PAIN: RECOMMENDED ACTIONS IN RESPONSE TO IMPORTANT HISTORICAL ELEMENTS
Source: **American College of Emergency Physicians**

	Actions[a]									
Character of Pain	A	B	C	D	E	F	G	H	I	J
1. Ongoing **and** severe **and** crushing **and** substernal **or** same as previous MI pain	++	++	+					+		
2. Severe or pressure or substernal or exertional or radiating to jaw, neck shoulder or arm	++	+	+					+		
3. Tearing, severe, and radiating to the back	++	++	++	+						
4. Similar to that of previous pulmonary embolus	++	++	+		++				+	
5. Indigestion or burning epigastric	+									
6. Pleuritic	+		+							
Patient Age										
7. Male > 33 years; female > 40 years	+									
Associated Symptoms										
8. Syncope or near syncope	++	+								3
9. SOB, DOE, PND, or orthopnea	++		+						+	
10. Significant hemoptysis			++						+	
11. Nausea/vomiting	+									
12. Productive or chronic cough										
13. Palpitations	+	+								
14. Significant weight change			+							
15. Diaphoresis	+									
Past Medical History										
16. Previous MI	++									
17. Coronary artery bypass graft/angioplasty	++									
18. Cocaine use within last 96 hours	++									1
19. Previous positive cardiac diagnostic studies	++									2
20. Cardiac medications (current)	+									1
21. Diuretics (current)										2
22. IV drug use (current)	+		+						+	

EVALUATING THE ADULT WITH ACUTE, NON-TRAUMATIC CHEST PAIN: RECOMMENDED ACTIONS IN RESPONSE TO IMPORTANT HISTORICAL ELEMENTS (CONTINUED)
Source: **American College of Emergency Physicians**

Character of Pain	Actions[a]									
	A	**B**	**C**	**D**	**E**	**F**	**G**	**H**	**I**	**J**
23. Major risk factors for coronary artery disease (a)	+									
24. Major risk factors for pulmonary embolus (b)	+		+		+	+			+	
25. Major risk factors for thoracic aortic aneurysm/dissection (c)	+		+	+						
26. Major risk factors for pericarditis/myocarditis (d)	+		+				+	+		
27. Major risk factors for pneumothorax (e)			+							
28. Major risk factors for pneumonia (f)			+						+	

++: An action reflecting principles of good practice in most situations. There may be circumstances when a rule need not or cannot be followed; in these situations, it is advisable that deviation from the rule be justified in writing.

+: An action that may be considered, depending on the patient, the circumstances, or other factors. Thus, these actions are not always followed, and there is no implication that failure to follow a guideline is improper.

[a]A = ECG; B = cardiac monitor; C = CXR; D = aortic imaging; E = pulmonary vasculature imaging; F = venous imaging; G = echocardiography; H = cardiac serum markers; I = ABG and/or oximetry; J = other testing (see footnotes).

(a) Coronary artery disease risk factors include: family hx; men age > 45 yrs, women age > 55 yrs; diabetes; hypertension; cigarette use; left ventricular hypertrophy; elevated cholesterol levels; hx chronic cocaine use.

(b) Pulmonary embolus risk factors include: prolonged immobilization; surgery > 30 min within past 3 months; hx deep venous thrombosis or pulmonary embolism; malignancy; pregnancy or recent pregnancy; hx of pelvis or lower extremity trauma; oral contraceptive use plus cigarette use; CHF; COPD; obesity; hypercoagulable state

(c) Thoracic aortic aneurysm/dissection risk factors include: hypertension; congenital disease of aorta or aortic valve; inflammatory disease of the aorta; connective tissue disease; pregnancy; arteriosclerosis; cigarette use

(d) Pericarditis/myocarditis risk factors include: infections (eg, tuberculosis, viral); autoimmune/ systematic disease (eg, lupus); acute rheumatic fever; recent MI or cardiac surgery; malignancy; radiation therapy to mediastinum; uremia; drugs (procainamide, hydralazine, INH, etc); hx of prior pericarditis

(e) Pneumothorax risk factors include: hx of previous pneumothorax; Valsalva maneuver; lung disease (obstructive, cancer, infection, connective tissue disease); cigarette use

(f) Pneumonia risk factors include: chronic lung disease; altered consciousness/impaired gag reflex; neuromuscular disease; thoracic cage deformity; cigarette use; preceding viral respiratory infection; immunodeficiency

1. Measurement of appropriate serum drug levels should be considered.
2. Measurement of K+ and Mg++ serum levels should be considered.
3. Measurement of the hematocrit should be considered.

Source: Modified from American College of Emergency Physicians: Clinical policy for the initial approach to adults presenting with a chief complaint of chest pain, with no history of trauma. Ann Emerg Med 1995;25:274–299.

EVALUATING THE ADULT WITH ACUTE, NON-TRAUMATIC CHEST PAIN: RECOMMENDED ACTIONS IN RESPONSE TO IMPORTANT PHYSICAL EXAMINATION FINDINGS
Source: **American College of Emergency Physicians**

	Actions[a]									
Vital Signs	**A**	**B**	**C**	**D**	**E**	**F**	**G**	**H**	**I**	**J**
1. Irregular pulse	+	++								
2. Tachypnea (RR > 24)	+								+	
3. Fever (> 38°C/100.4°F)			+							
4. Hypertension (SBP > 160 and/or DBP > 110)	+		+							
5. Tachycardia (> 100)	+								+	
6. Bradycardia (< 60)	+									
Appearance										
7. Cyanosis with respiratory distress	++	++	++		+				++	4
8. Diaphoresis	++		+					+	+	
Cardiovascular Exam										
9. Significant differences in right and left arm BPs	++	+	++	+						
10. New murmur	++		+				+			
11. Pericardial rub	++		+				+	+		
12. Irregular rhythm	+	++								
13. Jugular venous distention	+		+							
14. Third heart sound	+		+							
Pulmonary Exam										
15. Unilateral diminished breath sounds			++						+	
16. Localized dullness to percussion			+							
17. Pleural rub	+		+						+	
18. Unilateral rales			+						+	
19. Bilateral rales	+		+						+	
20. Wheezing	+	++	+						+	5
21. Unilateral leg swelling, pain, tenderness, warmth, erythema	+		+		+	+			+	
22. Bilateral edema	+		+							

EVALUATING THE ADULT WITH ACUTE, NON-TRAUMATIC CHEST PAIN: RECOMMENDED ACTIONS IN RESPONSE TO IMPORTANT PHYSICAL EXAMINATION FINDINGS (CONTINUED)
Source: American College of Emergency Physicians

++: An action reflecting principles of good practice in most situations. There may be circumstances when a rule need not or cannot be followed; in these situations, it is advisable that deviation from the rule be justified in writing.

+: An action that may be considered, depending on the patient, the circumstances, or other factors. Thus, these actions are not always followed, and there is no implication that failure to follow a guideline is improper.

[a]A = ECG; B = cardiac monitor; C = CXR; D = aortic imaging; E = pulmonary vasculature imaging; F = venous imaging; G = echocardiography; H = cardiac serum markers; I = ABG and/or oximetry; J = other testing (see footnotes).

4. Consider methemoglobin level and intubation.
5. Consider spirometry and bendrodilator therapy.

Source: Modified from American College of Emergency Physicians: Clinical policy for the initial approach to adults presenting with a chief complaint of chest pain, with no history of trauma. Ann Emerg Med 1995;25:274–299.

DEPRESSION: MANAGEMENT

OVERVIEW OF TREATMENT FOR DEPRESSION
Source: AHRQ

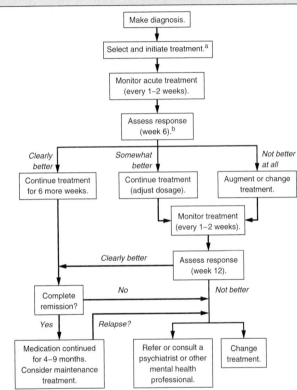

[a]ACP guidelines recommend that in patients with acute major depression or dysthmia, including elderly persons without significant comorbid conditions, consider either tricyclic antidepressants or newer antidepressants, such as selective serotonin reuptake inhibitors, as equally efficacious. For short-term treatment of mild acute depression, St. John's wort may be considered. However, patients should be cautioned that this treatment is not approved by the FDA, and preparations may vary substantially from those tested in randomized trials. (Ann Intern Med 2000;132:738)

[b]Times of assessment (weeks 6 and 12) rest on very modest data. It may be necessary to revise the treatment plan earlier for patients who fail to respond at all.

Source: Reproduced, with permission, from the AHRQ: Depression in Primary Care. Vol. 2: Treatment of Major Depression. United States Department of Health and Human Services, 1993.

DIABETES MELLITUS: MANAGEMENT

MANAGEMENT OF HYPERGLYCEMIA[a]
Source: ADA

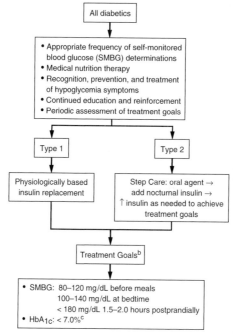

All diabetics

- Appropriate frequency of self-monitored blood glucose (SMBG) determinations
- Medical nutrition therapy
- Recognition, prevention, and treatment of hypoglycemia symptoms
- Continued education and reinforcement
- Periodic assessment of treatment goals

Type 1

Type 2

Physiologically based insulin replacement

Step Care: oral agent → add nocturnal insulin → ↑ insulin as needed to achieve treatment goals

Treatment Goals[b]

- SMBG: 80–120 mg/dL before meals
  100–140 mg/dL at bedtime
  < 180 mg/dL 1.5–2.0 hours postprandially
- HbA$_{1c}$: < 7.0%[c]

[a]Adapted from American Diabetes Association Position Statement Standards of Medical Care for Patients With Diabetes Mellitus. Last updated January 2003. (http://www.diabetes.org/DiabetesCare)

[b]These are generalized goals. They do not apply to pregnant adults. One should modify individual treatment goals to take into account risk for hypoglycemia, very young or old age, end-stage renal disease, advanced cardiovascular or cerebrovascular disease, or other diseases that decrease life expectancy.

[c]Based on results of the Diabetes Control and Complications Trial (DCCT) (Type 1) and the United Kingdom Prospective Diabetes Study (UKPDS) (Type 2).

Source: ADA Diabetes Care 2003;26(Suppl 1).

DIABETES MELLITUS: PREVENTION AND TREATMENT OF DIABETIC COMPLICATIONS

Source: ADA

PREVENTION & TREATMENT OF DIABETIC COMPLICATIONS

Complication	Goal	Monitoring/Treatment	Action if Goal Not Met
Hyperglycemia[a]	$HbA_{1c} < 7.0\%$[b] Preprandial plasma glucose 90–130 mg/dL Peak postprandial plasma glucose < 180 mg/dL	HbA_{1c} = every 6 months if meeting treatment goals; every 3 months in those not meeting goals.	See management, previous page
Retinopathy	Prevent vision loss	Annual retinal exam[c]	Laser treatment
Neuropathy	Prevent foot complications	Annual foot exam[d]	Examine feet at every visit; refer high-risk patients to a foot care specialist.
Nephropathy	Prevent renal failure	Annual urinary protein determination (see next page). Spot albumin: creatinine testing preferred.	See below[e]
Hypertension	Adult: BP < 130/80[f] mm Hg	Every routine diabetes visit	See JNC VII, page 127. If ACEs or adrenergic receptor binders are used, monitor renal function and potassium levels.
Hyperlipidemia	LDL < 100 mg/dL TG < 150 mg/dL HDL > 40 mg/dL	Annual determination, and more frequently to achieve goals. If low-risk (LDL < 100, HDL > 60, TG < 150), then assess every 2 years.	Weight loss; increase in physical activity; nutrition therapy; follow NCEP recommendations for pharmacologic treatment, Appendix VII

DIABETES MELLITUS: PREVENTION AND TREATMENT OF DIABETIC COMPLICATIONS
Source: ADA

PREVENTION & TREATMENT OF DIABETIC COMPLICATIONS (CONTINUED)

Complication	Goal	Monitoring/Treatment	Action if Goal Not Met
Macrovascular disease	Prevent stroke and MI	(1) Consider aspirin therapy as primary prevention for all patients ≥ 40 years and ≥ 1 cardiovascular risk factor. (2) Smoking cessation. (3) Manage hyperlipidemia and hypertension as above.	

[a]Less intensive glycemic goals if severe or frequent hypoglycemia.

[b]Postprandial glucose may be targeted if HbA1c goals are not met despite meeting preprandial goals.

[c]Dilated eye exam or 7-field 30-degree fundus photography by ophthalmologist or optometrist.

[d]Includes evaluation of protective sensation (monofilament test and tuning fork), vascular status, and inspection for foot deformities or ulcers.

[e]Microalbuminuria treatment: if type 1: ACE inhibitor; if type 2: individualize decision. Clinical albuminuria treatment: (1) Achieve BP < 130/80 mm Hg; (2) use ACE inhibitor or ARB; (3) tight glycemic control; and (4) decrease protein to 10% of dietary intake, especially in patients progressing despite optimal glucose and BP control. Refer to nephrologist if: estimated glomerular filtration rate < 30 mg/min, creatinine > 2.0 mg/dL, or when management of hypertension or hyperkalemia is difficult.

[f]ACP recommends tight BP control (SBP < 135, DBP < 80). ALLHAT trial showed no difference in cardiovascular and renal outcomes in diabetes treated with diuretics or ACE (or ARB). (JAMA 2002;288:2981) Diuretics should be first line in black patients. (Ann Intern Med 2003;138:587)

Source: Adapted from American Diabetes Association Position Statement "Standards of Medical Care for Patients With Diabetes Mellitus." Last updated January 2003. (http://www.diabetes.org/DiabetesCare)

PREVENTION & TREATMENT OF DIABETIC COMPLICATIONS (CONTINUED)

DIABETES MELLITUS: PREVENTION AND TREATMENT OF DIABETIC COMPLICATIONS
Source: ADA

| Category | Albuminuria Thresholds | | |
	24-hr collection (mg/24 hr)	Timed collection (µg/min)	Spot collection (albumin:creatinine ratio) (µg/mg)[a]
Normal	< 30	< 20	< 30
Microalbuminuria	30–299	20–200	30–299
Clinical (macro) albuminuria	≥ 300	> 200	≥ 300

Because of variability in urinary albumin excretion, 2 of 3 specimens collected within a 3- to 6-month period should be abnormal before considering a patient to have crossed one of these diagnostic thresholds. Exercise within 24 hours, infection, fever, congestive heart failure, marked hyperglycemia, and marked hypertension may elevate urinary albumin excretion over baseline values.

[a]Strongly encouraged as preferred test.

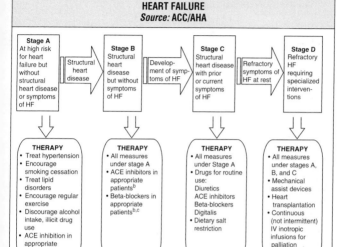

HEART FAILURE
Source: ACC/AHA

Stage A At high risk for heart failure but without structural heart disease or symptoms of HF	**Stage B** Structural heart disease but without symptoms of HF	**Stage C** Structural heart disease with prior or current symptoms of HF	**Stage D** Refractory HF requiring specialized interventions

Structural heart disease → / Development of symptoms of HF → / Refractory symptoms of HF at rest →

THERAPY
- Treat hypertension
- Encourage smoking cessation
- Treat lipid disorders
- Encourage regular exercise
- Discourage alcohol intake, illicit drug use
- ACE inhibition in appropriate patients[a]

THERAPY
- All measures under stage A
- ACE inhibitors in appropriate patients[b]
- Beta-blockers in appropriate patients[b,c]

THERAPY
- All measures under Stage A
- Drugs for routine use:
  Diuretics
  ACE inhibitors
  Beta-blockers
  Digitalis
- Dietary salt restriction

THERAPY
- All measures under stages A, B, and C
- Mechanical assist devices
- Heart transplantation
- Continuous (not intermittent) IV inotropic infusions for palliation
- Hospice care

Stage A: Patients with hypertension, coronary artery disease, diabetes mellitus *or* those using cardiotoxins or having a FHx CM

Stage B: Patients with previous MI, LV systolic dysfunction, or asymptomatic valvular disease

Stage C: Patients with known structural heart disease; shortness of breath and fatigue, reduced exercise tolerance

Stage D: Patients who have marked symptoms at rest despite maximal medical therapy (eg, those who are recurrently hospitalized or cannot be safely discharged from hospital without specialized interventions)

Footnotes:

[a] Appropriate patients include those with a history of atherosclerotic vascular disease, diabetes mellitus, or hypertension and associated cardiovascular risk factors.

[b] Appropriate patients for either ACE inhibitors or beta-blockers include those with recent or remote MI, regardless of ejection fraction; and those with reduced ejection fraction.

[c] Compared with placebo, beta-blocker use is associated with a consistent 30% reduction in mortality and 40% reduction in hospitalizations in patients with class II and III heart failure. (JAMA 2002;287:883)

Comments: Implementing a CHF disease management program for patients with ejection fractions < 20% was associated with decreased hospitalizations. (Arch Intern Med 2001;161:2223)

FHx CM = family history of cardiomyopathy; HF = heart failure; LV = left ventricle

Source: Adapted and reproduced with permission from the American College of Cardiology and American Heart Association, Inc. J Am Coll Cardiol 2001;38:2101.

HORMONE REPLACEMENT THERAPY

RISKS AND BENEFITS OF HORMONE REPLACEMENT THERAPY

	Risk for Untreated Women (Average)	Risk/Benefit with HRT
Breast Cancer	Lifetime risk 10%	An estrogen-progestin regimen (increased RR = 0.12/year of treatment) increases breast cancer risk beyond that associated with estrogen alone (increased RR = 0.03/year of treatment) among women with BMI ≤ 24.4 kg/m^2 (JAMA 2000;283:485). Incidence of breast cancer increased by 60%–85% in recent long-term users of HRT (> 5 years). (JAMA 2002;287:734–741) WHI: In intention-to-treat analysis, estrogen plus progestin increased total (hazard ratio, 1.24; 95% confidence interval, 1.02–1.50) and invasive (hazard ratio, 1.24; 95% confidence interval, 1.01–1.54) breast cancer. The increased risk of breast cancer with combined HRT appears to be independent of whether the progestin was taken in sequential or continuous manner. (JAMA 2003;289:3254–3263)
Coronary Heart Disease	46% lifetime probability of developing and 31% risk of dying from CHD After age 60 years, CHD is the primary cause of death for women.	HERS trial: showed no benefit of HRT on CHD events in women with a history of CAD (ie, secondary prevention). (JAMA 1998;280:605) HRT does not appear to reduce the risk of cardiovascular events in women with established CHD. Postmenopausal women without CHD: may be a slight increase in MI, strokes, thromboembolic events during first 1–2 years in HRT. (NEJM 2001;345:34–40) AHA: HRT should not be initiated for secondary prevention of CHD in postmenopausal women. (Circulation 2001;104:499–503) WHI: Combined HRT was associated with an increased risk for CHD (RR, 1.29; 95% confidence interval, 1.02–1.63; 29% increased risk). Elevation in risk most apparent at 1 year. (NEJM 2003;349:523–534)
Dementia	In North America, 7%–8% of persons 75–84 years of age have dementia.	WHI: Estrogen plus progestin therapy increased the risk for probable dementia in postmenopausal women aged ≥ 65 years (hazard ratio, 2.05; 95% confidence interval, 1.21–3.48; 45 vs 22 per 10,000 person-years; p = 0.01). (JAMA 2003;289:2651–2662) Estrogen plus progestin did not improve cognitive function when compared with placebo. (JAMA 2003;289:2663–2671)

	RISKS AND BENEFITS OF HORMONE REPLACEMENT THERAPY (CONTINUED)	
HORMONE REPLACEMENT THERAPY	
	Risk for Untreated Women (Average)	**Risk/Benefit with HRT**
Endometrial Cancer	Lifetime risk 2.6%	With unopposed estrogen, risk is increased 4- to 11-fold. Addition of progestins for at least 10 days per month prevents development of the endometrial hyperplasia associated with unopposed estrogen use. WHI: Nonsignificant decreased risk among women on estrogen plus progestin therapy (RR, 0.83; 95% confidence interval, 0.47–1.47). (JAMA 2002;288:321–333)
Stroke	Lifetime risk 20%	WHI: Estrogen plus progestin increases the risk of ischemic stroke in generally healthy postmenopausal women (hazard ratio, 1.44; 95% confidence interval, 1.09–1.90; 41% increased risk). (JAMA 2003;289:2673–2684)
Colorectal Cancer	Lifetime risk 6%	WHI: Significant decreased risk among women on estrogen plus progestin therapy (relative risk 0.63, 95% confidence interval 0.43–0.92, 37% decreased risk). (NEJM 2003;348:645–650)
Osteoporosis	15% lifetime probability of hip fracture (for white women)	Definite increase in BMD (2%–5%). Rates of vertebral, wrist, and hip fractures can be reduced by 25%–50% after 6–10 years of therapy (observational studies). *Data from randomized trials regarding effect of estrogen therapy on fractures are limited.
Ovarian Cancer		Estrogen-only HRT for ≥ 10 years is associated with 7% ↑ relative risk of ovarian cancer. (JAMA 2002;288:334–341)

HORMONE REPLACEMENT THERAPY

The USPSTF recommends against the routine use of estrogen and progestin for the prevention of chronic conditions in postmenopausal women. The USPSTF concluded that the harmful effects of estrogen and progestin are likely to exceed the chronic disease prevention benefits in most women. The USPSTF did not evaluate the use of HRT to treat symptoms of menopause, such as urogenital or vasomotor symptoms. The USPSTF concludes that the evidence is insufficient to recommend for or against the use of unopposed estrogen for the prevention of chronic conditions in postmenopausal women who have had a hysterectomy. (Ann Intern Med 2002;137:834–839)

Indications for Hormone Replacement Therapy: relief of menopausal symptoms (hot flushes, sweats, insomnia, vaginal dryness, pain with intercourse, recurrent UTIs). (NEJM 2003;348:1835–1837, NEJM 2003;348:579–580)

"When counseling women about HRT, consider the unique needs of each patient, and weigh benefits and risks on an individual basis." (JAMA 2002;288:368–369)

Alternatives to estrogen for treatment of menopausal symptoms: soy, isoflavones, St. John's wort, black cohosh, SSRIs. (www.acog.org, ACOG Practice Bulletin, June 2001) (NEJM 2001;345:34–40).

Women's Health Initiative has found overall health risks exceeded benefits from use of combined estrogen/progestin (0.625 mg/2.5 mg) for average 5.2 years follow-up. Risks included ↑ risk CHD, stroke, and pulmonary embolism beginning with treatment initiation, ↑ risk breast cancer after 5 years of therapy (0.38% per year breast cancer rate with HRT vs. 0.30% per year w/o HRT). (JAMA 2002;288:321–333)

Source: Ann Intern Med 1992;117:1016–1037, Ann Intern Med 2002;137:834–839, Menopause 2003;10:6–12.

HYPERTENSION: INITIATING TREATMENT
Source: The 7th Report of the Joint National Committee on Prevention, Detection,
Evaluation and Treatment of High Blood Pressure

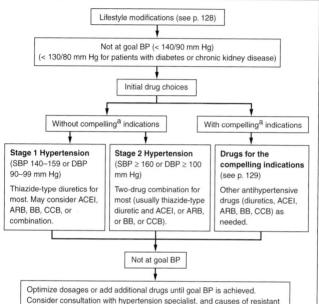

Lifestyle modifications (see p. 128)

Not at goal BP (< 140/90 mm Hg)
(< 130/80 mm Hg for patients with diabetes or chronic kidney disease)

Initial drug choices

Without compelling[a] indications

With compelling[a] indications

Stage 1 Hypertension
(SBP 140–159 or DBP
90–99 mm Hg)

Thiazide-type diuretics for
most. May consider ACEI,
ARB, BB, CCB, or
combination.

Stage 2 Hypertension
(SBP ≥ 160 or DBP ≥ 100
mm Hg)

Two-drug combination for
most (usually thiazide-type
diuretic and ACEI, or ARB,
or BB, or CCB).

**Drugs for the
compelling indications**
(see p. 129)

Other antihypertensive
drugs (diuretics, ACEI,
ARB, BB, CCB) as
needed.

Not at goal BP

Optimize dosages or add additional drugs until goal BP is achieved.
Consider consultation with hypertension specialist, and causes of resistant
hypertension (see p. 130).

Drug abbreviations: ACEI, ACE inhibitor; ARB, angiotensin receptor blocker; BB,
beta-blocker; CCB, calcium channel blocker.
[a]Compelling indications: CHF, high coronary disease risk, diabetes, chronic kidney
disease, recurrent stroke prevention.
Source: JNC VII, 2003.

LIFESTYLE MODIFICATIONS FOR PRIMARY PREVENTION OF HYPERTENSION[a,b]

Modification	Recommendation	Approximate SBP Reduction (Range)
Weight reduction	Maintain normal body weight (BMI 18.5–24.9 kg/m^2).	5–20 mm Hg per 10 kg weight loss
Adopt DASH eating plan	Consume diet rich in fruits, vegetables, and low fat dairy products with a reduced content of saturated and total fat.	8–14 mm Hg
Dietary sodium reduction	Reduce dietary sodium intake to no more than 100 mmol per day (2.4 g sodium or 6 g sodium chloride).	2–8 mm Hg
Physical activity	Engage in regular aerobic physical activity such as brisk walking (at least 30 min/day, most days of the week).	4–9 mm Hg
Moderation of alcohol consumption	Limit consumption to no more than 2 drinks (1 oz or 30 mL ethanol; eg, 24 oz beer, 10 oz wine, or 3 oz 80-proof whiskey) per day in most men and to no more than 1 drink per day in women and lighter weight persons.	2–4 mm Hg

DASH, Dietary Approaches to Stop Hypertension.
[a]For overall cardiovascular risk reduction, stop smoking.
[b]The effects of implementing these modifications are dose and time dependent and could be greater for some individuals.

RECOMMENDED MEDICATIONS FOR COMPELLING INDICATIONS						
	Recommended Medications[a]					
Compelling indication[b]	**Diuretic**	**BB**	**ACEI**	**ARB**	**CCB**	**AldoANT**
Heart failure	X	X	X	X		X
Post-MI		X	X			X
High coronary disease risk	X	X	X		X	
Diabetes	X	X	X	X	X	
Chronic kidney disease			X	X		
Recurrent stroke prevention	X		X			

[a]Drug abbreviations: ACEI, ACE inhibitor; ARB, angiotensin receptor blocker; AldoANT, aldosterone antagonist; BB, beta-blocker; CCB, calcium channel blocker.
[b]Compelling indications for antihypertensive drugs are based on benefits from outcome studies or existing clinical guidelines; the compelling indication is managed in parallel with the BP.

CAUSES OF RESISTANT HYPERTENSION
Improper BP Measurement
Volume Overload and Pseudotolerance
Excess sodium intake
Volume retention from kidney disease
Inadequate diuretic therapy
Drug-Induced or Other Causes
Nonadherence
Inadequate doses
Inappropriate combinations
Nonsteroidal anti-inflammatory drugs; cyclooxygenase 2 inhibitors
Cocaine, amphetamines, other illicit drugs
Sympathomimetics (decongestants, anoretics)
Oral contraceptives
Adrenal steroids
Cyclosporine and tacrolimus
Erythropoietin
Licorice (including some chewing tobacco)
Select over-the-counter dietary supplements and medicines (eg, ephedra, mahaung, bitter orange)
Associated Conditions
Obesity
Excess alcohol intake
Identifiable Causes
Sleep apnea
Chronic kidney disease
Primary aldosteronism
Renovascular disease
Steroid excess
Pheochromocytoma
Coarctation of aorta
Thyroid or parathyroid disease

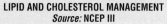

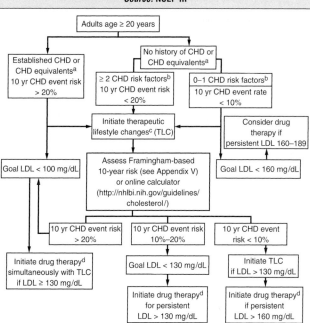

LIPID AND CHOLESTEROL MANAGEMENT
Source: NCEP III

[a]CHD risk equivalents carry a risk for major coronary events equal to that of established CHD (ie, > 20% per 10 years), and include: diabetes, other clinical forms of arthrosclerotic disease (peripheral arterial disease, abdominal aortic aneurysm, and symptomatic carotid artery disease).

[b]Age (men ≥ 45 years, women ≥ 55 years or postmenopausal), hypertension (BP ≥ 140/90 mm Hg or on antihypertensive medication), cigarette smoking, HDL < 40 mg/dL, family history of premature CHD in first-degree relative (males < 55 years, females < 65 years). Diabetes now considered CHD risk equivalent. For HDL ≥ 60 mg/dL, subtract 1 risk factor from above.

[c]All patients, particularly those with elevated cholesterol levels, should be encouraged to adopt the following lifestyle changes: reduce saturated fat (< 7% total calories) and cholesterol (< 200 mg/d intake; increase physical activity; and achieve appropriate weight control (see publication for greater details on TLC regimens). Assess effects of TLC on lipid levels after 3 months.

[d]Drug therapy response should be monitored and modified at 6-week intervals to achieve goal LDL levels; after goal LDL met, monitor response and adherence every 4–6 months.

Source: Executive summary of the third report of the National Cholesterol Education Project (NCEP) expert panel on detection, evaluation and treatment of high blood cholesterol in adults (Adult Treatment Panel III). JAMA 2001;285:2486.

ADULT ACUTE LOW BACK PAIN: ALGORITHM 1. INITIAL EVALUATION
Sources: Agency for Healthcare Research and Quality; American Academy
of Family Practitioners; American College of Radiology,
American Academy of Orthopedic Surgeons

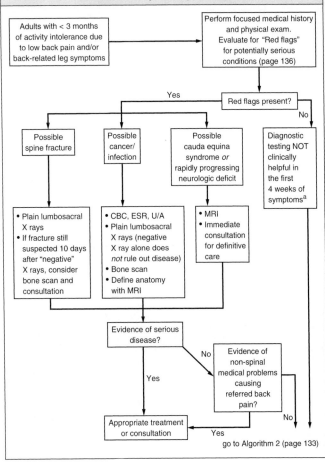

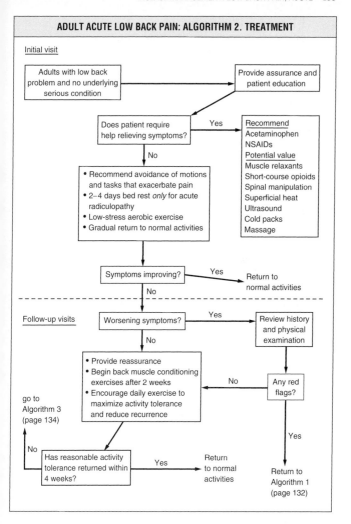

ADULT ACUTE LOW BACK PAIN: ALGORITHM 2. TREATMENT

Initial visit

Adults with low back problem and no underlying serious condition → Provide assurance and patient education

Does patient require help relieving symptoms? — Yes → Recommend Acetaminophen / NSAIDs / Potential value Muscle relaxants / Short-course opioids / Spinal manipulation / Superficial heat / Ultrasound / Cold packs / Massage

No ↓

• Recommend avoidance of motions and tasks that exacerbate pain
• 2–4 days bed rest *only* for acute radiculopathy
• Low-stress aerobic exercise
• Gradual return to normal activities

↓

Symptoms improving? — Yes → Return to normal activities

No ↓

Follow-up visits

Worsening symptoms? — Yes → Review history and physical examination

No ↓

• Provide reassurance
• Begin back muscle conditioning exercises after 2 weeks
• Encourage daily exercise to maximize activity tolerance and reduce recurrence

← No — Any red flags?

Yes ↓

go to Algorithm 3 (page 134)

No ↑

Has reasonable activity tolerance returned within 4 weeks? — Yes → Return to normal activities

Return to Algorithm 1 (page 132)

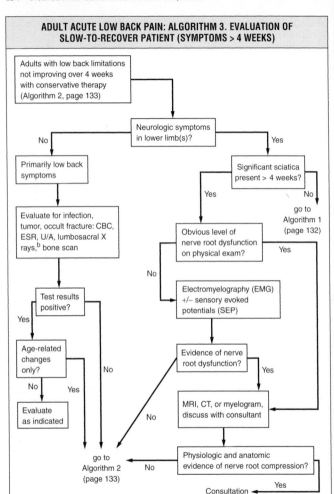

ADULT ACUTE LOW BACK PAIN: ALGORITHM 3. EVALUATION OF SLOW-TO-RECOVER PATIENT (SYMPTOMS > 4 WEEKS)

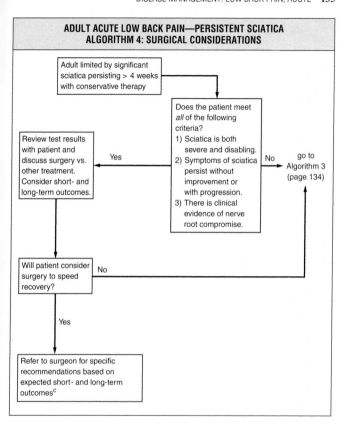

ADULT ACUTE LOW BACK PAIN—PERSISTENT SCIATICA
ALGORITHM 4: SURGICAL CONSIDERATIONS

Adult limited by significant sciatica persisting > 4 weeks with conservative therapy

Does the patient meet *all* of the following criteria?
1) Sciatica is both severe and disabling.
2) Symptoms of sciatica persist without improvement or with progression.
3) There is clinical evidence of nerve root compromise.

Yes → Review test results with patient and discuss surgery vs. other treatment. Consider short- and long-term outcomes.

No → go to Algorithm 3 (page 134)

Will patient consider surgery to speed recovery?

No →

Yes ↓

Refer to surgeon for specific recommendations based on expected short- and long-term outcomes[c]

RED FLAGS FOR POTENTIALLY SERIOUS CONDITIONS			
History Features	**Fracture**	**Cancer or Infection**	**Cauda Equina Syndrome**
Major trauma, ie, motor vehicle accident or fall from height	×		
Minor trauma or strenuous lifting (older or osteoporotic patient)	×		
Age > 50 or < 20		×	
History of cancer		×	
Constitutional symptoms (ie, fever, weight loss)		×	
Risk factors for spinal infection (ie, recent bacterial infection, IV drug use, immune suppression)		×	
Pain that worsens when supine		×	
Severe nighttime pain		×	
Saddle anesthesia			×
Recent onset of bladder dysfunction (ie, urinary retention, increased frequency, overflow incontinence)			×
Severe or progressive lower extremity neurologic deficit			×
Physical Examination Features			
Anal sphincter laxity			×
Perianal/perineal sensory loss			×
Major motor weakness: knee extension, foot drop			×

Footnotes for Adult Acute Low Back Pain Algorithms

[a]Footnote to Algorithm 1:

It has generally been believed that 80%–90% of acute low back pain episodes recover spontaneously within 4 weeks. However, more recent studies indicate that there may be a significant percentage of individuals who continue to have pain or functional limitation at 1 year. Recurrences are common, affecting 40% of patients within 6 months. The emerging picture is that of a chronic problem with intermittent exacerbations, rather than an acute disease that can be cured.

Sources:

Atlas SI, Deyo RA. Evaluating and managing acute low back pain in the primary care setting. J Gen Intern Med 2001;16:120–131.

Deyo RA, Weinstein JM. Low back pain. NEJM 2001;244:363–370.

Cherkin DC, Deyo RA, Street JH, Barlow W. Predicting poor outcomes for back pain seen in primary care using patients' own reports. Spine 1966;21:2900–2907.

Croft PR, Macfarlane GJ, Papageorgiou AC, et al. Outcome of low back pain in general practice: a prospective study. BMJ 1998;316:1356–1359.

Thomas E, Silman AJ, Croft PR, et al. Predicting who develops chronic low back pain in primary care: a prospective study. BMJ 1999;318:1662–1667.

[b]Footnote to Algorithm 3:

In an RCT, MRIs and radiographs resulted in nearly identical outcomes for primary care patients with low back pain. Substituting MRI for radiographs in the primary care setting may offer little additional benefit to patients and may increase the cost of care. (JAMA 2003;289:2810–2818)

[c]Footnote to Algorithm 4:

Herniated disk: Surgery for herniated disks is invasive and comprises all types of surgical and injection techniques to remove or reduce the size of herniated intervertebral disks that compress nerve roots. Included are standard discectomy, microscopic discectomy, percutaneous discectomy, and chemonucleolysis. The therapeutic objective is to relieve pressure on nerve roots and reduce pain and possibly weakness and/or numbness in the lower extremities. Lumbar discectomy may relieve symptoms faster than continued nonsurgical therapy in patients who have severe and disabling leg symptoms and who have not improved after 4–8 weeks of adequate nonsurgical treatment. However, in nonemergent patients, there appears to be little difference in long-term outcomes at 4 and 10 years between discectomy and conservative care.

Spinal stenosis: Elderly patients with spinal stenosis who can adequately function in the activities of daily life can be managed with conservative treatments. Surgery for spinal stenosis should not usually be considered in the first 3 months of symptoms. Decisions on treatment should take into account the patient's lifestyle, preference, other medical problems, and risk of surgery. In one study of patients with severe lumbar spinal stenosis, surgical treatment was associated with greater improvement in patient-reported outcomes than nonsurgical treatment at 4 years (70% vs 52% reported that their predominant symptom was better). The relative benefit of surgery declined over time but remained superior to nonsurgical treatment. (Atlas SJ, Keller RB, Robson D, Deyo RA, Singer DE. Surgical and nonsurgical management of lumbar spinal stenosis: four-year outcomes from the Maine Lumbar Spine Study. Spine 2000;25:556–62)

Sources:

Bigos S et al. Acute low back problems in adults. Rockville, MD: U.S. Department of Health and Human Services, Public Health Service, Agency for Health Care Policy and Research, 1994. AHCPR Publication no. 95-0642.

Patel AT, Oble AA. Diagnosis and Management of Acute Low Back Pain. Am Fam Physician 2000;61:1779–86. American College of Radiology. ACR Appropriateness Criteria. www.acr.org. (website accessed 10/18/03); American Academy of Orthopedic Surgeons Clinical Guideline on Low Back Pain (www.aaos.org, website accessed 10/18/03).

OBESITY MANAGEMENT: ADULTS
Source: NHLBI

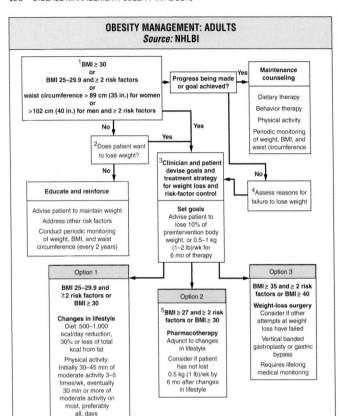

Notes for Obesity Management Guideline: Adults

1. Risk factors: cigarette smoking; hypertension or current use of antihypertensive agents; LDL cholesterol ≥ 160 mg/dL or LDL cholesterol 130–159 mg/dL+ ≥ 2 other risk factors; HDL cholesterol < 35 mg/dL; fasting plasma glucose 110–125 mg/dL; family history of premature CHD (MI or sudden death in 1st degree ♂ relative ≤ 55 years old or 1st degree ♀ relative ≤ 65 years old; age ≥ 45 for ♂ or ≥ 55 years for ♀.

2. The decision to lose weight must be made in the context of other risk factors (eg, quitting smoking is more important than losing weight).

3. The decision to lose weight must be made jointly between the clinician and the patient.

4. Investigate: patient's level of motivation; energy intake (dietary recall); energy expenditure (physical activity diary); attendance at psychological/behavioral counseling sessions; recent negative life events; family and societal pressures; evidence of detrimental psychiatric problems (eg, depression, binge eating disorder).

5. Pharmacotherapy should be considered as an adjunct only for patients who are at substantial medical risk because of their obesity and in whom nonpharmacologic treatments have not resulted in sufficient weight loss to improve health. The safety and efficacy of weight-loss medications beyond 2 years of use have not been established. Two medications available for long-term use; sibutramine (5–15 mg/day) and/or orlistat (120 mg 3 times/day with or within 1 hour after fat-containing meals, plus a daily multivitamin).

Source: Adapted from the National Institutes of Health. NEJM 2002;346[8]:591–599; http://www.nhlbi.nih.gov/guidelines/obesity/ob_home.htm

OBESITY MANAGEMENT: CHILDREN
Source: **Expert Committee, Department of Health and Human Services**

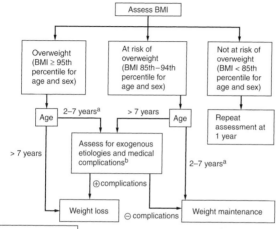

Approach to therapy:

1. Begin interventions early—risk of persistent obesity increases with age of child.
2. Family must be ready to change—defer treatment until family ready or refer to therapist.
3. Educate families about medical complications of obesity.
4. Involve family and *all* caregivers in treatment program.
5. Institute permanent changes—methodic, gradual, long-term changes will be more successful than multiple, frequent changes.
6. Family should learn to monitor eating and activity.
7. Recommend 2–3 specific changes in diet or activity at a time—additional recommendations only after success.
8. Emphasize successful behavior changes rather than weight loss; empathize with struggles experienced.
9. Utilize a team approach; consider group meetings.
10. Provide guidance in parenting skills—avoid using food as a reward; offer only healthy options; be a role model.
11. Increase activity level: limit television, incorporate activity into usual daily activities, aim for ≥ 30 minutes of activity on most days.
12. Reduce calorie intake: identify and eliminate high-calorie foods.
13. Stop tobacco use (adolescents).

Footnotes:

[a] Children younger than 2 years should be referred to a pediatric obesity center.
[b] Evaluate for: 1. <u>Exogenous causes</u>: genetic syndromes, hypothyroidism, Cushing's syndrome, eating disorders, depression; 2. <u>Complications</u>: hypertension, dyslipidemias, noninsulin-dependent diabetes mellitus, slipped capital femoral epiphysis, pseudotumor cerebri, sleep apnea or obesity hypoventilation syndrome, gallbladder disease, polycystic ovary disease.

Source: Pediatrics 1998;102(3) (www.pediatrics.org/cgi/content/full/102/3/e29)

OSTEOPOROSIS: MANAGEMENT[c]
Source: American Academy of Clinical Endocrinologists

Known osteoporotic fracture or osteoporosis by DXA[a]

Treatment for all:
- Calcium supplementation 1,000–1,500 mg/day
- Vitamin D 400–800 IU/day
- Weight-bearing exercise 30 min/day, 3 d/wk
- Avoid heparin
- Avoid glucocorticoids

+

Pharmacologic Management[b]

Agents approved for treatment of osteoporosis:
- Bisphosphonates (alendronate, risedronate)
  - ↑ BMD of spine, hip and ↓ vertebral and nonvertebral fracture risk
- Calcitonin
  - ↓ vertebral but *not* nonvertebral fracture risk
  - modest ↑ spinal BMD
  - analgesic effect in acute osteoporotic fracture
- Estrogen (see HRT table, page 124)
  - Given increased risks of other outcomes demonstrated in the Women's Health Initiative (WHI), must individualize risk/benefit assessment.
  - ↓ vertebral and hip fracture risk
- Selective estrogen receptor modulators (SERMs—Raloxifene)
  - Modest ↑ BMD spine and hip
  - ↓ vertebral fracture risk
  - No documented ↓ in nonvertebral fracture risk
- Parathyroid Hormone (Forteo)
  - Subcutaneous injection
  - ↓ risk of vertebral and nonvertebral fractures
- Combination Therapy (bisphosphate + non-bisphosphate)
  - Can provide additional small ↑ BMD vs. monotherapy
  - Impact on fracture risk unknown

[a]Indications for treatment
- ♀ with T scores below –2 in the absence of risk factors
- ♀ with T scores below –1.5 if other risk factors present
- Age > 70 with multiple risk factors, even without BMD testing
- Prior vertebral or hip fracture

[b]Selection of pharmacologic agents for treating osteoporosis should be based on individual risk/benefit and preferences. Bisphosphanates are indicated for male osteoporosis and for glucocorticoid-induced osteoporosis.

[c]Follow-up: perform follow-up BMD yearly for 2 years. If bone mass stabilizes after 2 years, remeasure every 2 years. Otherwise, continue annual BMD until bone mass is stable. Medicare covers BMD every 2 years. Biochemical markers of BME turnover can be used to monitor response to treatment.

Source: Adapted from AACE 2001 Medical Guidelines for Clinical Practice for the Prevention and Management of Postmenopausal Osteoporosis and NOF guidelines for treatment (www.nof.org, website accessed 10/18/03).

PAP SMEAR ABNORMALITIES: MANAGEMENT AND FOLLOW-UP[a]

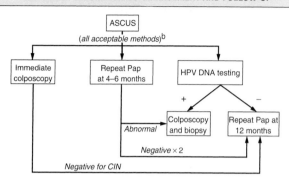

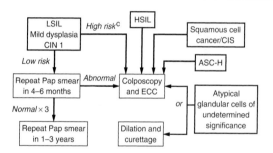

[a] Assumes satisfactory specimen; if unsatisfactory, repeat Pap smear. If no endocervical cells, follow-up in 1 year for low risk with previously negative smear, repeat in 4–6 mo. for high risk.

[b] Postmenopausal women: provide a course of intravaginal estrogen followed by repeat Pap smear 1 week after completing therapy. If repeat Pap negative, repeat in 4–6 months. If negative × 2, return to routine screening. If repeat test ASCUS or greater, refer for colposcopy. Immunosuppressed women should have immediate referral to colposcopy.

[c] High risk: history of abnormal Pap smear, high-risk HPV DNA, unlikely to return for follow-up.

ASCUS = atypical squamous cells of undetermined significance; ECC = endocervical curettage; LSIL = low-grade squamous intraepithelial lesion; CIN = cervical intraepithelial neoplasia; HSIL = high-grade squamous intraepithelial lesion; CIS = carcinoma in situ. ASC-H = atypical squamous cells, cannot exclude HSIL.

If endometrial cells are found in women aged ≥ 40 years, perform endometrial biopsy.

Source: Modified from JAMA 2002;287:2120–2129, Up-to-Date: Management of the abnormal Papanicolaou smear (www.uptodate.com, accessed 10/18/03).

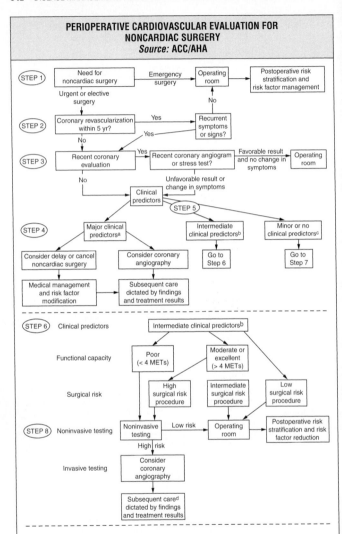

PERIOPERATIVE CARDIOVASCULAR EVALUATION FOR NONCARDIAC SURGERY
Source: ACC/AHA

PERIOPERATIVE CARDIOVASCULAR EVALUATION FOR NONCARDIAC SURGERY (CONTINUED)
Source: ACC/AHA

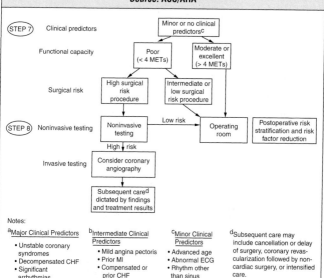

Notes:

[a]Major Clinical Predictors

- Unstable coronary syndromes
- Decompensated CHF
- Significant arrhythmias
- Severe valvular disease

[b]Intermediate Clinical Predictors

- Mild angina pectoris
- Prior MI
- Compensated or prior CHF
- Diabetes mellitus
- Renal insufficiency

[c]Minor Clinical Predictors

- Advanced age
- Abnormal ECG
- Rhythm other than sinus
- Low functional capacity
- History of stroke
- Uncontrolled systemic hypertension

[d]Subsequent care may include cancellation or delay of surgery, coronary revascularization followed by non-cardiac surgery, or intensified care.

Source: Adapted from Eagle KA, Berger PB, Calkins H, et al. ACC/AHA guideline update for perioperative cardiovascular evaluation for noncardiac surgery update: a report of the American College of Cardiology/American Heart Association Task Force on Practice Guidelines (Committee to Update the 1996 Guidelines on Perioperative Cardiovascular Evaluation for Noncardiac Surgery). 2002. American College of Cardiology website. Available at: http://www.acc.org/clinical/guidelines/perio/update/periupdate_index.htm

COMMUNITY-ACQUIRED PNEUMONIA
Source: ATS

Group I	Group II	Group IIIa	Group IIIb
Outpatient No cardiopulm Hx[a] No modifying factors[b]	Outpatient w/ cardiopulm Hx[a] or modifiers[b]	Inpatients Not ICU No cardiopulm Hx[a] No modifying factors[b]	Inpatients Not ICU w/ cardiopulm Hx[a] or modifiers[b]
↓	↓	↓	↓
Azithromycin/ Clarithromycin or Doxycycline	Beta-Lactam *plus* Macrolide or doxycycline *OR* Fluoroquinolone[c]	IV azithromycin or Fluoroquinolone[c]	IV Beta-Lactam *plus* IV or oral macrolide or doxycycline *OR* Fluoroquinolone[c]

[a]Such as chronic obstructive pulmonary disease or congestive heart failure.

[b]Presence of risk factors for drug-resistant pneumococcus (aged > 65 yr, beta-lactam therapy within past 3 mo, alcoholism, immunosuppression, multiple medical comorbidities, exposure to child in day care center) presence of risk factors for gram negative infection (residence in nursing home, cardiopulmonary disease multiple medical comorbidities, recent antibiotic therapy), and risk factors for *Pseudomonas aeruginosa* [structural lung disease, corticosteroid therapy (>10 mg prednisone per day), broad spectrum antibiotic therapy for > 7 d past month, malnutrition].

[c]Use fluoroquinolone with anti-streptococcus pneumonia activity.

Source: Modified from Am J Resp Crit Care Med 2001;163:1730–1754.

APPROACH TO COUGH ILLNESS (BRONCHITIS) IN ADULTS
Source: CDC

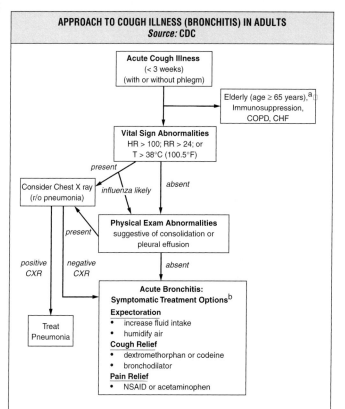

[a]Pneumonia in the elderly, as well as those with comorbidity, often presents atypically. Evaluation should be individualized.

[b]If duration of illness is > 2 weeks, consider pertussis. PCR or culture testing for pertussis is done to confirm the diagnosis and indicate the need for public health follow-up to prevent illness among contacts, especially infants. Antibiotic therapy can decrease shedding, but has no effect on symptoms during the paroxysmal phase (≥ 10 days after illness onset). Treat with erythromycin × 14 days pending results.

Source: Adapted from Centers for Disease Control and Prevention; Ann Intern Med 2001; 134:521.

APPROACH TO ACUTE SORE THROAT (PHARYNGITIS) IN ADULTS
Source: CDC

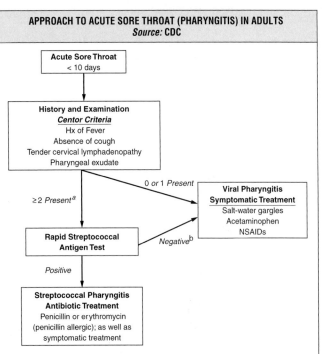

[a]Acceptable alternatives to these strategies include: 1) test and treat patients with 2 or 3 Centor criteria present, and empirically treat with antibiotics (do not test) patients with 4 Centor criteria; or 2) do not test any patients, and empirically treat with antibiotics patients with 3 or 4 Centor criteria present.

[b]Do not recommend culture-confirmation of negative rapid antigen tests in adults when the sensitivity of the rapid antigen test exceeds 80%. When performed in adults with ≥ 2 criteria present, the sensitivity exceeds 90%. (Ann Emerg Med 2001;38:648)

These principles apply to immunocompetent adults without complicated comorbidities such as chronic lung or heart disease, history of rheumatic fever, or during known group A streptococcal outbreaks. They also are not intended to apply during a known epidemic of acute rheumatic fever or streptococcal pharyngitis, or for nonindustrialized countries where the endemic rate of acute rheumatic fever is much higher than it is in the U.S.

Source: Adapted from Centers for Disease Control and Prevention; Ann Intern Med 2001; 134:509.

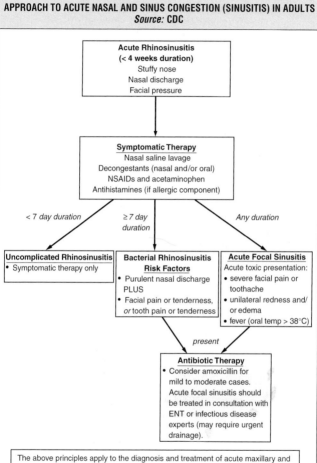

APPROACH TO ACUTE NASAL AND SINUS CONGESTION (SINUSITIS) IN ADULTS
Source: CDC

Acute Rhinosinusitis
(< 4 weeks duration)
Stuffy nose
Nasal discharge
Facial pressure

↓

Symptomatic Therapy
Nasal saline lavage
Decongestants (nasal and/or oral)
NSAIDs and acetaminophen
Antihistamines (if allergic component)

< 7 day duration   *≥7 day duration*   *Any duration*

Uncomplicated Rhinosinusitis
• Symptomatic therapy only

Bacterial Rhinosinusitis
Risk Factors
• Purulent nasal discharge
  PLUS
• Facial pain or tenderness,
  or tooth pain or tenderness

Acute Focal Sinusitis
Acute toxic presentation:
• severe facial pain or
  toothache
• unilateral redness and/
  or edema
• fever (oral temp > 38°C)

present

Antibiotic Therapy
• Consider amoxicillin for
  mild to moderate cases.
  Acute focal sinusitis should
  be treated in consultation with
  ENT or infectious disease
  experts (may require urgent
  drainage).

The above principles apply to the diagnosis and treatment of acute maxillary and ethmoid rhinosinusitis in non-immunocompromised adults.

Source: Adapted from Centers for Disease Control and Prevention; Ann Intern Med 2001; 134:498.

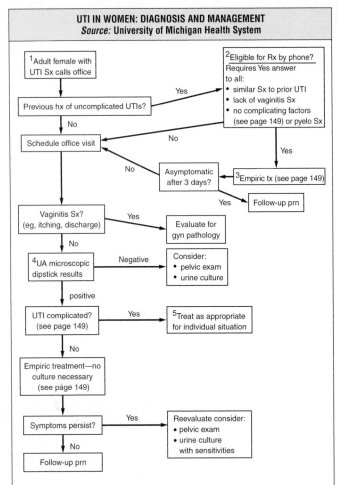

UTI IN WOMEN: DIAGNOSIS AND MANAGEMENT
Source: University of Michigan Health System

[1]Adult female with UTI Sx calls office

Previous hx of uncomplicated UTIs?

[2]Eligible for Rx by phone?
Requires Yes answer to all:
• similar Sx to prior UTI
• lack of vaginitis Sx
• no complicating factors (see page 149) or pyelo Sx

Yes

No

Schedule office visit

Yes

Asymptomatic after 3 days?

[3]Empiric tx (see page 149)

Yes

Follow-up prn

No

Vaginitis Sx? (eg, itching, discharge)

Yes → Evaluate for gyn pathology

No

[4]UA microscopic dipstick results

Negative → Consider:
• pelvic exam
• urine culture

positive

UTI complicated? (see page 149)

Yes → [5]Treat as appropriate for individual situation

No

Empiric treatment—no culture necessary (see page 149)

Symptoms persist?

Yes → Reevaluate consider:
• pelvic exam
• urine culture with sensitivities

No

Follow-up prn

Source: Adapted from University of Michigan Health System, Urinary Tract Infection guideline, June 1999; Infectious Diseases Society of America (IDSA) practice guideline (Clinical Infectious Diseases 1999;29:745–758); Am J Med 1999;106:636–641; NEJM 2003;349:259–266.

UTI IN WOMEN ALGORITHM, NOTES AND TABLES

LABORATORY CHARGES AND RELATIVE COSTS

Test	Relative Cost
Urinalysis, dipstick	$
Urinalysis, complete microscopic	$$
Urine culture	$$$

COMPLICATING FACTORS

- Catheter
- Diabetes mellitus
- Immunosuppression
- Nephrolithiasis
- Pregnancy
- Pyelonephritis symptoms
- Recent hospitalization or nursing home residence
- Recurrent UTIs (> 3/year)
- Symptoms for > 7 days
- Urologic structural/functional abnormality

TREATMENT REGIMENS AND RELATIVE COSTS

Treatment Regimen	Relative Cost
First Line	
Trimethoprim/Sulfa DS BID × 3 days	$
Second Line (in preferred order)	
Trimethoprim 100 mg TID × 3 days	$
Ciprofloxacin 100 mg BID × 3 days	$$
Norfloxacin 400 mg BID × 3 days	$$$
Ofloxacin 200 mg BID × 3 days	$$$
Amoxicillin 500 mg TID × 7 days	$$
Nitrofurantoin 100 mg QID × 7 days	$$$$
Nitrofurantoin 100 mg BID × 7 days	$$$

1. The majority of UTIs occur in sexually active women. Risk increases by 3–5 times when diaphragms are used for contraception. Risk also increases slightly with not voiding after sexual intercourse and use of spermicides. Dysuria with either urgency or frequency, in the absence of vaginal symptoms, yields a prior probability of UTI of 70%–80%. Generally, UTI symptoms are of abrupt onset (< 3 days).

2. The majority of UTIs in women are uncomplicated and resolve readily with brief courses of antibiotics. Therefore, many women can be assessed and safely managed without an office visit or laboratory examination. A study of a telephone-based clinical practice guideline for managing presumed uncomplicated cystitis among women aged 18–55 years found that guideline implementation significantly decreased the proportion of patients with presumed cystitis who received urinalysis, urine culture, or an initial office visit. The guideline also increased the proportion of women who received a guideline-recommended antibiotic. Adverse outcomes (return office visit, sexually transmitted disease, pyelonephritis within 60 days of initial diagnosis) did not increase as a result of guideline implementation. The study authors concluded that guideline use decreased laboratory utilization and overall costs while maintaining or improving the quality of care for patients who were presumptively treated for acute uncomplicated cystitis. (Saint S, Scholes D, Fihn S, Farrell R, Stamm W. The effectiveness of a clinical practice guideline for the management of presumed uncomplicated urinary tract infection in women. Am J Med 1999;106:636–641)

3. Acute uncomplicated cystitis in women traditionally has been treated with longer (7–10 day) courses of antibiotics. More recent studies have found shorter courses (3–5 days) of oral antibiotics to be as effective as traditional courses. A review of 28 treatment trials of adult women with uncomplicated cystitis concluded that no benefit was achieved by increasing the length of therapy beyond 5 days. (Norrby SR. Short-term treatment of uncomplicated lower urinary tract infections in women. Rev Infect Dis 1990;12:458–467) The optimal treatment of uncomplicated UTI in patients who are not allergic or sensitive is 3 days of TMP/SMX.

4. Dipstick analysis for leukocyte esterase, an indirect test for the presence for pyuria, is the least expensive and least time-intensive diagnostic test for UTI. It is estimated to have a sensitivity of 75%–96% and specificity of 94%–98%. Nitrite testing by dipstick is less useful, in large part because it is only positive in the presence of bacteria that produce nitrate reductase, and can be confounded by consumption of ascorbic acid. Microscopic examination of unstained, centrifuged urine by a trained observer under $40 \times$ power has a sensitivity of 82%–97% and a specificity of 84%–95%. For urine culture, sensitivity varies from 50%–95%, depending on the threshold for UTI, and specificity varies from 85%–99%. Because of the limited sensitivity of urine culture, and the delay required for results, urine culture is not recommended to diagnose or verify uncomplicated UTI.

5. Unlike women with uncomplicated UTI, care for women with complicating factors includes:
   - Culture: Obtain pretreatment culture and sensitivity.
   - Treatment: Initiate treatment with trimethoprim/sulfa or quinolone for 7–14 days (quinolones contraindicated in pregnancy).
   - Follow-up UA: Obtain follow-up urinalysis to document clearing.
   - Possible structural evaluation: Lower threshold for urologic structural evaluation with cysto/IVP.

4
Appendices

	SCREENING INSTRUMENTS: ALCOHOL ABUSE

SENSITIVITY AND SPECIFICITY OF SCREENING TESTS FOR PROBLEM DRINKING

Instrument Name	Screening Questions/Scoring	Threshold Score	Sensitivity/Specificity (%)	Source
CAGE[a]	See page 153	> 1 > 2 > 3	77/58 53/81 29/92	Am J Psychiatr 1974;131:1121 J Gen Intern Med 1998;13:379
AUDIT	See page 153	> 4 > 5 > 6	87/70 77/84 66/90	BMJ 1997;314:420 J Gen Intern Med 1998;13:379

[a]The CAGE may be less applicable to binge drinkers (eg, college students), the elderly, and minority populations.

SCREENING INSTRUMENTS: ALCOHOL ABUSE

SCREENING PROCEDURES FOR PROBLEM DRINKING

1. CAGE screening test[a]

Have you ever felt the need to	Cut down on drinking?.
Have you ever felt	Annoyed by criticism of your drinking?.
Have you ever felt	Guilty about your drinking?.
Have you ever taken a morning	Eye opener?

INTERPRETATION: Two "yes" answers are considered a positive screen. One "yes" answer should arouse a suspicion of alcohol abuse.

2. The alcohol use disorder identification test (AUDIT).[b] (Scores for response categories are given in parentheses. Scores range from 0 to 40, with a cutoff score of ≥ 5 indicating hazardous drinking, harmful drinking, or alcohol dependence.)

1 How often do you have a drink containing alcohol?

(0) Never   (1) Monthly or less   (2) Two to four times a month   (3) Two or three times a week   (4) Four or more times a week

2 How many drinks containing alcohol do you have on a typical day when you are drinking?

(0) 1 or 2   (1) 3 or 4   (2) 5 or 6   (3) 7 to 9   (4) 10 or more

3 How often do you have six or more drinks on one occasion?

(0) Never   (1) Less than monthly   (2) Monthly   (3) Weekly   (4) Daily or almost daily

4 How often during the past year have you found that you were not able to stop drinking once you had started?

(0) Never   (1) Less than monthly   (2) Monthly   (3) Weekly   (4) Daily or almost daily

5 How often during the past year have you failed to do what was normally expected of you because of drinking?

(0) Never   (1) Less than monthly   (2) Monthly   (3) Weekly   (4) Daily or almost daily

SCREENING INSTRUMENTS: ALCOHOL ABUSE

SCREENING PROCEDURES FOR PROBLEM DRINKING (CONTINUED)

6 How often during the past year have you needed a first drink in the morning to get yourself going after a heavy drinking session?

(0) Never   (1) Less than monthly   (2) Monthly   (3) Weekly   (4) Daily or almost daily

7 How often during the past year have you had a feeling of guilt or remorse after drinking?

(0) Never   (1) Less than monthly   (2) Monthly   (3) Weekly   (4) Daily or almost daily

8 How often during the past year have you been unable to remember what happened the night before because you had been drinking?

(0) Never   (1) Less than monthly   (2) Monthly   (3) Weekly   (4) Daily or almost daily

9 Have you or has someone else been injured as a result of your drinking?

(0) No   (2) Yes, but not in the past year   (4) Yes, during the past year

10 Has a relative or friend or a doctor or other health worker been concerned about your drinking or suggested you cut down?

(0) No   (2) Yes, but not in the past year   (4) Yes, during the past year

[a]Modified from Mayfield D et al. The CAGE questionnaire: Validation of a new alcoholism screening instrument. Am J Psychiatry 1974;131:1121.
[b]From Piccinelli M et al. Efficacy of the alcohol use disorders identification test as a screening tool for hazardous alcohol intake and related disorders in primary care: A validity study. BMJ 1997;314:420.

SCREENING INSTRUMENTS: COGNITIVE IMPAIRMENT

THE ANNOTATED MINI MENTAL STATE EXAMINATION (AMMSE)

MiniMental LLC

Suspect dementia when score ≤ 24.

NAME OF SUBJECT _____ Age _____

NAME OF EXAMINER _____ Years of School Completed ___

Approach the patient with respect and encouragement. Date of Examination _____

Ask: Do you have any trouble with your memory? ☐ Yes ☐ No

May I ask you some questions about your memory? ☐ Yes ☐ No

SCORE ITEM

5 ( ) **TIME ORIENTATION**

Ask:

What is the year _____ (1), season _____ (1),

month of the year _____ (1), date _____ (1),

day of the week _____ (1)?

5 ( ) **PLACE ORIENTATION**

Ask:

Where are we now? What is the state _____ (1), city _____ (1),

part of the city _____ (1), building _____ (1),

floor of the building _____ (1)?

3 ( ) **REGISTRATION OF THREE WORDS**

Say: Listen carefully. I am going to say three words. You say them back after I stop.

Ready? Here they are...PONY (wait 1 second), QUARTER (wait 1 second), ORANGE

(wait 1 second). What were those words?

_____ (1)

_____ (1)

_____ (1)

Give 1 point for each correct answer, then repeat them until the patient learns all three.

5 ( ) **SERIAL 7s AS A TEST OF ATTENTION AND CALCULATION**

Ask: Subtract 7 from 100 and continue to subtract 7 from each subsequent remainder

until I tell you to stop. What is 100 take away 7?_____ (1)

Say:

Keep going. _____ (1), _____ (1),

_____ (1), _____ (1).

3 ( ) **RECALL OF THREE WORDS**

Ask:

What were those three words I asked you to remember?

Give one point for each correct answer. _____ (1),

_____ (1), _____ (1),

2 ( ) **NAMING**

Ask:

What is this? (show pencil) _____ (1). What is this? (show watch) _____ (1).

For more

information or

additional copies

of this exam,

call (617)587-4215

© 1975, 1998 MiniMental LLC

SCREENING INSTRUMENTS: COGNITIVE IMPAIRMENT

MiniMental LLC

1 ( ) **REPETITION**
Say:
Now I am going to ask you to repeat what I say. Ready? No ifs, ands or buts.
Now you say that. _____ (1)

3 ( ) **COMPREHENSION**
Say:
Listen carefully because I am going to ask you to do something.
Take this paper in your left hand (1), fold it in half (1), and put it on the floor. (1)

1 ( ) **READING**
Say:
Please read the following and do what it says, but do not say it aloud. (1)

Close your eyes

1 ( ) **WRITING**
Say:
Please write a sentence. If the patient does not respond, say: Write about the weather. (1)
_____
_____

1 ( ) **DRAWING**
Say: Please copy this design.

TOTAL SCORE _____ Assess level of consciousness along a continuum

Alert	Drowsy	Stupor	Coma

	YES	NO			YES	NO	FUNCTION BY PROXY
Cooperative:	☐	☐	Deterioration from				Please record date when patient was last able to perform the following tasks. Ask caregiver if patient independently handles:
Depressed:	☐	☐	previous level of				
Anxious:	☐	☐	functioning:		☐	☐	
Poor Vision:	☐	☐	Family History of Dementia:	☐	☐		YES NO DATE
Poor Hearing:	☐	☐	Head Trauma:		☐	☐	Money/Bills: ☐ ☐ _____
Native Language:			Stroke:		☐	☐	Medication: ☐ ☐ _____
_____			Alcohol Abuse:		☐	☐	Transportation: ☐ ☐ _____
			Thyroid Disease:		☐	☐	Telephone: ☐ ☐ _____

Source: Reproduced with permission from "Mini-Mental State." A practical method for grading the cognitive state of patients for the clinician. J Psychiatr Res 1975;12(3):189.
©1975, 1998 MiniMental LLC.

SCREENING INSTRUMENTS: DEPRESSION

SCREENING TESTS FOR DEPRESSION

Instrument Name	Screening Questions/Scoring	Threshold Score	Source
Beck Depression Inventory (Short Form)	See page 158	0–4: none or minimal depression 5–7: mild depression 8–15: moderate depression > 15 = severe depression	Postgrad Med 1972;Dec:81
Geriatric Depression Scale	See page 158	≥ 15 = depression	J Psychiatr Res 1983;17:37
PRIME-MD© (mood questions)	(1) During the past month, have you often been bothered by feeling down, depressed, or hopeless? (2) During the past month, have you often been bothered by little interest or pleasure in doing things?	"Yes" to either question[a]	JAMA 1994;272:1749 J Gen Intern Med 1997;12:439

[a]Sensitivity 86%–96%, specificity 57%–75%.
©Pfizer Inc.

SCREENING INSTRUMENTS: DEPRESSION

BECK DEPRESSION INVENTORY, SHORT FORM

Instructions: This is a questionnaire. On the questionnaire are groups of statements. Please read the entire group of statements in each category. Then pick out the one statement in that group that best describes the way you feel today, that is, *right now!* Circle the number beside the statement you have chosen. If several statements in the group seem to apply equally well, circle each one. Sum all numbers to calculate a score.

Be sure to read all the statements in each group before making your choice.

A. Sadness
3 I am so sad or unhappy that I can't stand it.
2 I am blue or sad all the time and I can't snap out of it.
1 I feel sad or blue.
0 I do not feel sad.

B. Pessimism
3 I feel that the future is hopeless and that things cannot improve.
2 I feel I have nothing to look forward to.
1 I feel discouraged about the future.
0 I am not particularly pessimistic or discouraged about the future.

C. Sense of failure
3 I feel I am a complete failure as a person (parent, husband, wife).
2 As I look back on my life, all I can see is a lot of failures.
1 I feel I have failed more than the average person.
0 I do not feel like a failure.

D. Dissatisfaction
3 I am dissatisfied with everything.
2 I don't get satisfaction out of anything anymore.
1 I don't enjoy things the way I used to.
0 I am not particularly dissatisfied.

E. Guilt
3 I feel as though I am very bad or worthless.
2 I feel quite guilty.
1 I feel bad or unworthy a good part of the time.
0 I don't feel particularly guilty.

F. Self-dislike
3 I hate myself.
2 I am disgusted with myself.
1 I am disappointed in myself.
0 I don't feel disappointed in myself.

G. Self-harm
3 I would kill myself if I had the chance.
2 I have definite plans about committing suicide.
1 I feel I would be better off dead.
0 I don't have any thoughts of harming myself.

H. Social withdrawal
3 I have lost all of my interest in other people and don't care about them at all.
2 I have lost most of my interest in other people and have little feeling for them.
1 I am less interested in other people than I used to be.
0 I have not lost interest in other people.

I. Indecisiveness
3 I can't make any decisions at all anymore.
2 I have great difficulty in making decisions.
1 I try to put off making decisions.
0 I make decisions about as well as ever.

J. Self-image change
3 I feel that I am ugly or repulsive-looking.
2 I feel that there are permanent changes in my appearance and they make me look unattractive.
1 I am worried that I am looking old or unattractive.
0 I don't feel that I look any worse than I used to.

SCREENING INSTRUMENTS: DEPRESSION

BECK DEPRESSION INVENTORY, SHORT FORM (CONTINUED)

K. Work difficulty
3 I can't do any work at all.
2 I have to push myself very hard to do anything.
1 It takes extra effort to get started at doing something.
0 I can work about as well as before.

L. Fatigability
3 I get too tired to do anything.
2 I get tired from doing anything.
1 I get tired more easily than I used to.
0 I don't get any more tired than usual.

M. Anorexia
3 I have no appetite at all anymore.
2 My appetite is much worse now.
1 My appetite is not as good as it used to be.
0 My appetite is no worse than usual.

Source: Reproduced with permission from Beck AT, Beck RW. Screening depressed patients in family practice: A rapid technic. Postgrad Med 1972;52:81.

GERIATRIC DEPRESSION SCALE

Choose the best answer for how you felt over the past week

1. Are you basically satisfied with your life?	yes / no
2. Have you dropped many of your activities and interests?	yes / no
3. Do you feel that your life is empty?	yes / no
4. Do you often get bored?	yes / no
5. Are you hopeful about the future?	yes / no
6. Are you bothered by thoughts you can't get out of your head?	yes / no
7. Are you in good spirits most of the time?	yes / no
8. Are you afraid that something bad is going to happen to you?	yes / no
9. Do you feel happy most of the time?	yes / no
10. Do you often feel helpless?	yes / no
11. Do you often get restless and fidgety?	yes / no
12. Do you prefer to stay at home, rather than going out and doing new things?	yes / no
13. Do you frequently worry about the future?	yes / no
14. Do you feel you have more problems with memory than most?	yes / no
15. Do you think it is wonderful to be alive now?	yes / no

SCREENING INSTRUMENTS: DEPRESSION

GERIATRIC DEPRESSION SCALE (CONTINUED)

16. Do you often feel downhearted and blue?	yes / no
17. Do you feel pretty worthless the way you are now?	yes / no
18. Do you worry a lot about the past?	yes / no
19. Do you find life very exciting?	yes / no
20. Is it hard for you to get started on new projects?	yes / no
21. Do you feel full of energy?	yes / no
22. Do you feel that your situation is hopeless?	yes / no
23. Do you think that most people are better off than you are?	yes / no
24. Do you frequently get upset over little things?	yes / no
25. Do you frequently feel like crying?	yes / no
26. Do you have trouble concentrating?	yes / no
27. Do you enjoy getting up in the morning?	yes / no
28. Do you prefer to avoid social gatherings?	yes / no
29. Is it easy for you to make decisions?	yes / no
30. Is your mind as clear as it used to be?	yes / no

One point for each response suggestive of depression. (Specifically "no" responses to questions 1, 5, 7, 9, 15, 19, 21, 27, 29, and 30, and "yes" responses to the remaining questions are suggestive of depression.)

A score of ≥ 15 yields a sensitivity of 80% and a specificity of 100%, as a screening test for geriatric depression. Clin Gerontologist 1982;1:37.

Source: Reproduced with permission from Yesavage JA et al. Development and validation of a geriatric depression screening scale: A preliminary report. J Psychiatr Res 1982–83;17:37.

FUNCTIONAL ASSESSMENT SCREENING IN THE ELDERLY			
Target Area	**Assessment Procedure**	**Abnormal Result**	**Suggested Intervention**
Vision	Ask: "Do you have difficulty driving or watching television or reading or doing any of your daily activities because of your eyesight?" Test each eye with Jaeger card while patient wears corrective lenses (if applicable).	"Yes" and inability to read greater than 20/40	Refer to ophthalmologist.
Hearing	Whisper a short, easily answered question such as "What is your name?" in each ear while the examiner's face is out of direct view.	Inability to answer question	Examine auditory canals for cerumen and clean if necessary. Repeat test; if still abnormal in either ear, refer for audiometry and possible prosthesis.
Arm	Proximal: "Touch the back of your head with both hands." Distal: "Pick up the spoon."	Inability to do task	Examine the arm fully (muscle, joint, and nerve), paying attention to pain, weakness, limited range of motion. Consider referral for physical therapy.
Leg	Observe the patient after instructing as follows: "Rise from your chair, walk 10 feet, return, and sit down."	Inability to walk or transfer out of chair	Do full neurologic and musculoskeletal evaluation, paying attention to strength, pain, range of motion, balance, and gait. Consider referral for physical therapy.
Continence of urine	Ask, "Do you ever lose your urine and get wet?"	"Yes"	Ascertain frequency and amount. Search for remediable causes, including local irritations, polyuric states, and medications. Consider urologic referral.
Nutrition	Ask, "Without trying, have you lost 10 lb or more in the last 6 months?" Weigh the patient. Measure height.	"Yes" or weight is below acceptable range for height	Do appropriate medical evaluation.

FUNCTIONAL ASSESSMENT SCREENING IN THE ELDERLY (CONTINUED)			
Target Area	**Assessment Procedure**	**Abnormal Result**	**Suggested Intervention**
Mental status	Instruct as follows: "I am going to name three objects (pencil, truck, book). I will ask you to repeat their names now and then again a few minutes from now."	Inability to recall all three objects after 1 minute	Administer Folstein Mini-Mental State Examination. If score is less than 24, search for causes of cognitive impairment. Ascertain onset, duration, and fluctuation of overt symptoms. Review medications. Assess consciousness and affect. Do appropriate laboratory tests.
Depression	Ask, "Do you often feel sad or depressed?" or "How are your spirits?"	"Yes" or "Not very good, I guess"	Administer Geriatric Depression Scale. If positive (score above 15), check for antihypertensive, psychotropic, or other pertinent medications. Consider appropriate pharmacologic or psychiatric treatment.
ADL-IADL[a]	Ask, "Can you get out of bed yourself?" "Can you dress yourself?" "Can you make your own meals?" "Can you do your own shopping?"	"No" to any question	Corroborate responses with patient's appearance; question family members if accuracy is uncertain. Determine reasons for the inability (motivation compared with physical limitation). Institute appropriate medical, social, or environmental interventions.
Home environment	Ask, "Do you have trouble with stairs inside or outside of your home?" Ask about potential hazards inside the home with bathtubs, rugs, or lighting.	"Yes"	Evaluate home safety and institute appropriate countermeasures.

FUNCTIONAL ASSESSMENT SCREENING IN THE ELDERLY (CONTINUED)			
Target Area	**Assessment Procedure**	**Abnormal Result**	**Suggested Intervention**
Social support	Ask, "Who would be able to help you in case of illness or emergency?"	. . .	List identified persons in the medical record. Become familiar with available resources for the elderly in the community.

[a]Activities of daily living–instrumental activities of daily living.
Source: Modified from Lachs MS et al. A simple procedure for screening for functional disability in elderly patients. Ann Intern Med 1990;112:699.
Geriatrics at your fingertips online edition 2003 (www.geriatricsatyourfingertips.org, accessed 12/12/03).

95TH PERCENTILE OF BLOOD PRESSURE FOR BOYS

Age (y)	SBP (mm Hg) by percentile of height							DBP (mm Hg) by percentile of height						
	5%	10%	25%	50%	75%	90%	95%	5%	10%	25%	50%	75%	90%	95%
3	105	106	107	109	111	112	113	63	63	64	65	66	67	68
4	107	108	109	111	113	114	115	67	68	68	69	70	71	72
5	108	109	111	113	114	116	117	71	71	72	73	74	75	76
6	109	110	112	114	116	117	118	74	75	75	76	77	78	79
7	110	111	113	115	117	118	119	77	77	78	79	80	81	81
8	112	113	114	116	118	119	120	79	79	80	81	82	83	83
9	113	114	116	118	119	121	122	80	81	81	82	83	84	85
10	115	116	117	119	121	123	123	81	82	83	83	84	85	86
11	117	118	119	121	123	125	125	82	82	83	84	85	86	87
12	119	120	122	124	125	127	128	83	83	84	85	86	87	87
13	121	122	124	126	128	129	130	83	83	84	85	86	87	88
14	124	125	127	129	131	132	133	83	84	85	86	87	87	88
15	127	128	130	132	133	135	136	84	85	86	86	87	88	89
16	130	131	133	134	136	138	138	86	86	87	88	89	90	90
17	132	133	135	137	139	140	141	88	88	89	90	91	92	93

95TH PERCENTILE OF BLOOD PRESSURE FOR GIRLS

Age (y)	SBP (mm Hg) by percentile of height							DBP (mm Hg) by percentile of height						
	5%	10%	25%	50%	75%	90%	95%	5%	10%	25%	50%	75%	90%	95%
3	104	104	106	107	108	109	110	65	65	66	66	67	68	68
4	105	106	107	108	109	111	111	68	68	69	69	70	71	71
5	107	107	108	110	111	112	113	71	71	71	72	73	74	74
6	108	109	110	111	113	114	114	73	73	74	74	75	76	76
7	110	111	112	113	114	115	116	75	75	75	76	77	78	78
8	112	113	114	115	116	117	118	76	77	77	78	79	79	80
9	114	115	116	117	118	119	120	78	78	79	79	80	81	81
10	116	117	118	119	120	122	122	79	79	80	81	81	82	83
11	118	119	120	121	122	124	124	81	81	81	82	83	83	84
12	120	121	122	123	125	126	126	82	82	82	83	84	85	85
13	122	123	124	125	126	128	128	83	83	84	84	85	86	86
14	124	125	126	127	128	129	130	84	84	85	85	86	87	87
15	125	126	127	128	130	131	131	85	85	85	86	87	88	88
16	126	127	128	129	130	132	132	85	85	86	87	87	88	88
17	127	127	128	130	131	132	133	85	86	86	87	88	88	89

Source: Adapted with permission from Rosner B et al. Blood pressure nomograms for children and adolescents, by height, sex, and age, in the United States. J Pediatr 1993;123:874.

	BMI 25 kg/m²	BMI 27 kg/m²	BMI 30 kg/m²
BODY MASS INDEX CONVERSION TABLE			
Height in inches (cm)	Body weight in pounds (kg)		
58 (147.32)	119 (53.98)	129 (58.51)	143 (64.86)
59 (149.86)	124 (56.25)	133 (60.33)	148 (67.13)
60 (152.40)	128 (58.06)	138 (62.60)	153 (69.40)
61 (154.94)	132 (59.87)	143 (64.86)	158 (71.67)
62 (157.48)	136 (61.69)	147 (66.68)	164 (74.39)
63 (160.02)	141 (63.96)	152 (68.95)	169 (76.66)
64 (162.56)	145 (65.77)	157 (71.22)	174 (78.93)
65 (165.10)	150 (68.04)	162 (73.48)	180 (81.65)
66 (167.64)	155 (70.31)	167 (75.75)	186 (84.37)
67 (170.18)	159 (72.12)	172 (78.02)	191 (86.64)
68 (172.72)	164 (74.39)	177 (80.29)	197 (89.36)
69 (175.26)	169 (76.66)	182 (82.56)	203 (92.08)
70 (177.80)	174 (78.93)	188 (85.28)	207 (93.90)
71 (180.34)	179 (81.19)	193 (87.54)	215 (97.52)
72 (182.88)	184 (83.46)	199 (90.27)	221 (100.25)
73 (185.42)	189 (85.73)	204 (92.53)	227 (102.97)
74 (187.96)	194 (88.00)	210 (95.26)	233 (105.69)
75 (190.50)	200 (90.72)	216 (97.98)	240 (108.86)
76 (193.04)	205 (92.99)	221 (100.25)	246 (111.59)

Metric conversion formula = weight (kg)/height (m²)	**Non-metric conversion formula = [weight (pounds)/height (inches)²] × 704.5**
Example of BMI calculation:	Example of BMI calculation:
A person who weighs 78.93 kilograms and is 177 centimeters tall has a BMI of 25:	A person who weighs 164 pounds and is 68 inches (or 5' 8") tall has a BMI of 25:
weight (78.93 kg)/height (1.77 m)² = 25	[weight (164 pounds)/height (68 inches)²] × 704.5 = 25

Source: Adapted from NHLBI Obesity Guidelines in Adults, 1998.

ESTIMATE OF 10-YEAR CARDIAC RISK FOR MEN[a]

Age (y)	Points
20–34	−9
35–39	−4
40–44	0
45–49	3
50–54	6
55–59	8
60–64	10
65–69	11
70–74	12
75–79	13

Total Cholesterol	Points				
	Age 20–39	Age 40–49	Age 50–59	Age 60–69	Age 70–79
< 160	0	0	0	0	0
160–199	4	3	2	1	0
200–239	7	5	3	1	0
240–279	9	6	4	2	1
≥ 280	11	8	5	3	1

	Points				
	Age 20–39	Age 40–49	Age 50–59	Age 60–69	Age 70–79
Nonsmoker	0	0	0	0	0
Smoker	8	5	3	1	1

HDL (mg/dL)	Points
≥ 60	−1
50–59	0
40–49	1
< 40	2

Systolic BP (mm Hg)	If Untreated	If Treated
< 120	0	0
120–129	0	1
130–139	1	2
140–159	1	2
≥ 160	2	3

Point Total	10-Year Risk %	Point Total	10-Year Risk %
< 0	< 1	9	5
0	1	10	6
1	1	11	8
2	1	12	10
3	1	13	12
4	1	14	16
5	2	15	20
6	2	16	25
7	3	≥ 17	≥ 30
8	4		

10-Year risk_____%

[a]Framingham point scores.
Source: U.S. Department of Health and Human Services, Public Health Service, National Institutes of Health, National Heart, Lung, and Blood Institute.
NIH Publication No. 01-3305, May 2001.

ESTIMATE OF 10-YEAR CARDIAC RISK FOR WOMEN[a]

Age (y)	Points
20–34	−7
35–39	−3
40–44	0
45–49	3
50–54	6
55–59	8
60–64	10
65–69	12
70–74	14
75–79	16

Total Cholesterol	Age 20–39	Age 40–49	Points Age 50–59	Age 60–69	Age 70–79
< 160	0	0	0	0	0
160–199	4	3	2	1	1
200–239	8	6	4	2	1
240–279	11	8	5	3	2
≥ 280	13	10	7	4	2

	Age 20–39	Age 40–49	Points Age 50–59	Age 60–69	Age 70–79
Nonsmoker	0	0	0	0	0
Smoker	9	7	4	2	1

HDL (mg/dL)	Points
≥ 60	−1
50–59	0
40–49	1
< 40	2

Systolic BP (mmHg)	If Untreated	If Treated
< 120	0	0
120–129	1	3
130–139	2	4
140–159	3	5
≥ 160	4	6

Point Total	10-Year Risk %	Point Total	10-Year Risk %
< 9	< 1	17	5
9	1	18	6
10	1	19	8
11	1	20	11
12	1	21	14
13	2	22	17
14	2	23	22
15	3	24	27
16	4	≥ 25	≥ 30

10-Year risk _____%

[a]Framingham point scores.
Source: U.S. Department of Health and Human Services, Public Health Service, National Institutes of Health, National Heart, Lung, and Blood Institute.
NIH Publication No. 01-3305, May 2001.

PROFESSIONAL SOCIETIES & GOVERNMENTAL AGENCIES

Abbreviation	Full Name	Internet Address
AACE	American Association of Clinical Endocrinologists	www.aace.com
AAD	American Academy of Dermatology	www.aad.org
AAFP	American Academy of Family Physicians	www.aafp.org
AAO	American Academy of Ophthalmology	www.aao.org
AAOHNS	American Academy of Otolaryngology/ Head & Neck Surgery	www.entnet.org
AAOS	American Academy of Orthopedic Surgeons	www.aaos.org
AAP	American Academy of Pediatrics	www.aap.org
ACC	American College of Cardiology	www.acc.org
ACCP	American College of Chest Physicians	www.chestnet.org
ACIP	Advisory Committee on Immunization Practices	wonder.cdc.gov
ACOG	American College of Obstetricians and Gynecologists	www.acog.com
ACP	American College of Physicians	www.acponline.org
ACPM	American College of Preventive Medicine	www.acpm.org
ACR	American College of Radiology	www.acr.org
ACS	American Cancer Society	www.cancer.org
ACSM	American College of Sports Medicine	www.acsm.org
ADA	American Diabetes Association	www.diabetes.org
AGA	American Gastroenterological Association	www.gastro.org
AGS	American Geriatrics Society	www.americangeriatrics.org
AHA	American Heart Association	www.americanheart.org
AHRQ	Agency for Healthcare Research and Quality	www.ahrq.gov
AMA	American Medical Association	www.ama-assn.org
ANA	American Nurses Association	www.nursingworld.org
AOA	American Optometric Association	www.aoanet.org
ASCRS	American Society of Colon and Rectal Surgeons	www.fascrs.org

PROFESSIONAL SOCIETIES & GOVERNMENTAL AGENCIES (CONTINUED)

Abbreviation	Full Name	Internet Address
ASCO	American Society of Clinical Oncology	www.asco.org
ASGE	American Society for Gastrointestinal Endoscopy	www.asge.org
ASHA	American Speech-Language-Hearing Association	www.asha.org
ATA	American Thyroid Association	www.thyroid.org
ATS	American Thoracic Society	www.thoracic.org
AUA	American Urological Association	auanet.org
CDC	Centers for Disease Control and Prevention	www.cdc.gov
CNS	Canadian Neurological Society	www.ccns.org
CTF	Canadian Task Force on the Periodic Health Examination	www.ctfphc.org
GAPS	Guidelines for Adolescent Preventative Services	
NCI	National Cancer Institute	cancer.gov/cancerinformation
NEI	National Eye Institute	www.nei.nih.gov
NGC	National Guidelines Clearinghouse	www.guidelines.gov
NHLBI	National Heart, Lung, and Blood Institute	www.nhlbi.nih.gov
NIDR	National Institute of Dental and Craniofacial Research	www.nidr.nih.gov
NIHCDC	National Institutes of Health Consensus Development Conference	www.consensus.nih.gov
NIP	National Immunization Program	www.cdc.gov.nip
NOF	National Osteoporosis Foundation	www.nof.org
NTSB	National Transportation Safety Board	www.ntsb.gov
SCF	Skin Cancer Foundation	www.skincancer.org
SGIM	Society for General Internal Medicine	www.sgim.org
SVU	Society for Vascular Ultrasound	www.svunet.org
USPSTF	United States Preventive Services Task Force	www.ahrq.gov/clinic/uspstfix.htm

REFERENCES

The Canadian Task Force on the Periodic Health Examination: The Canadian Guide to Clinical Preventive Health Care. Minister of Public Works and Government Services Canada, 1994. (Referred to as "CTF" in tables). Updated guidelines available at: http://www.ctfphc.org.

Elster AB (ed): American Medical Association. AMA Guidelines for Adolescent Preventive Services (GAPS): Recommendations and Rationale. Williams & Wilkins, 1994. (Referred to as "GAPS" in tables)

Bright Futures: Guidelines for Health Supervision of Infants, Children, and Adolescents. Bright Futures at Georgetown University. 2nd ed, rev. 2002. (www.brightfutures.org) (Referred to as "Bright Futures" in tables)

U.S. Preventive Services Task Force: Guide to Clinical Preventive Services, 2nd ed. Williams & Wilkins, 1996. (Referred to as "USPSTF" in tables) Updated guidelines now available at http://www.ahcpr.gov/clinic/uspstfix.htm

Geriatrics at Your Fingertips. Blackwell Publishing, 2003. Online version: www.geriatricsatyourfingertips.org.

Index

A

Abuse
child, screening for, 33
domestic, screening for, 43
elder, screening for, 43
ACE inhibitors
in diabetes, 80
in heart failure, 123
in hypertension, 86, 127, 129
Acetaminophen
in acute cough, 145
in acute lower back pain, 133
in acute rhinosinusitis, 147
in arthritis, 98
in sore throat, 146
Acquired immunodeficiency syndrome (AIDS). See Human immunodeficiency virus (HIV)
Activities of daily living-instrumental activities of daily living (ADL-IADL), 162
Adolescents
blood pressure percentiles in
for boys, 164
for girls, 165
screening in
for abuse and neglect, 33
for alcohol abuse and dependence, 2
for cholesterol and lipid disorders, 35
for depression, 39
for hearing impairment, 46
for hypertension, 52
for iron-deficient anemia, 4
for scoliosis, 62
Advisory Committee on Childhood Lead Poisoning Prevention (ACCLPP), 55
AIDS. See Human immunodeficiency virus (HIV)

Albuminuria, in diabetic patients, 122
Alcohol abuse and dependence
screening for, 2–3
sensitivity and specificity of tests for, 152
tests for, 153–154
Alcohol Use Disorders Identification Test (AUDIT), 2, 153–154
Aldosterone antagonists, in hypertension, 129
Alendronate, in osteoporosis, 82, 140
Allergic rhinitis, 94–95
Alpha-1-antitrypsin deficiency, as risk factor for liver cancer, 20
Alphafetoprotein, in liver cancer screening, 20
Amblyopia, screening for, 68
Anemia, iron-deficient, screening for, 4
Angiotensin-converting enzyme (ACE) inhibitors
in diabetes, 80
in heart failure, 123
in hypertension, 86, 127, 129
Angiotensin receptor blockers, in hypertension, 127, 129
Annotated Mini Mental State Examination, 155–156
Antibiotics
in community-acquired pneumonia, 144
in endocarditis prevention, 75
in rhinosinusitis and sinusitis, 147
in streptococcal pharyngitis, 146
in urinary tract infections, 149
Anticholinergics, in allergic rhinitis, 95
Anticoagulation, and stroke prevention, 84
Antihistamines
in allergic rhinitis, 95
in nasal and sinus congestion, 147

Arthritis, of hip and knee, management of, 96–98
Aspirin, and stroke prevention, 84
Asthma
    severity classification of, 99–100
    treatment of, 101–105
Asymptomatic Carotid Artery Atherosclerosis Study (ACAS), 31
Atopic dermatitis, management of, 106–108
Atrial fibrillation
    evaluation and management algorithm for, 109–110
    and stroke prevention, 84, 85
Audiologic evaluations, 45–46, 161
AUDIT (Alcohol Use Disorders Identification Test), 2, 153–154

B
Back pain, acute low
    evaluation of, 137
    initial evaluation of, 132
    red flags for potentially serious conditions in, 136
    surgical considerations for, 135
    treatment of, 133
Barium enema, in colorectal cancer screening, 16
Beck Depression Inventory (Short Form), 40, 157–159
Beta$_2$-agonists, in asthma, 101–105
Beta blockers
    in heart failure, 123
    in hypertension, 127, 129
Bisphosphonates, in osteoporosis, 82, 140
Bladder cancer
    risk factors for, 5
    screening for, 5
Blood pressure (BP). *See also* Hypertension
    management of, 127
    percentiles in
        for boys, 164
        for girls, 165
    screening for, 52–54

Body mass index (BMI)
    conversion table for, 166
    in obesity screening, 57, 138–139
Bone mineral density (BMD), in osteoporosis screening, 58
Breast cancer
    CA-15-3, CEA in, 9
    hormone replacement therapy and, 124
    prevention of, 72–73
    risk factors for, 73
    screening for, 6–9, 72
Breast self-exam, in breast cancer screening, 6
Bronchitis, acute, evaluation and management of, 145
Bronchodilators
    in acute cough, 145
    in asthma, 101–105

C
CAGE test for alcoholism, 2, 152–153
Calcitonin, in osteoporosis, 140
Calcium channel blockers, in hypertension, 127, 129
Calcium supplementation, in osteoporosis, 140
Cardiac risk, 10-year, estimate of
    for men, 167
    for women, 168
Cardiovascular evaluation, perioperative, for noncardiac surgery, 142–143
Cardiovascular exam, in acute, nontraumatic chest pain, 116
Carotid artery stenosis (asymptomatic)
    management of, 111
    screening for, 31–32
    and stroke prevention, 85
Cataracts
    evaluation and management algorithm for, 112–113
    screening for, 68
CA-125 tumor marker, in ovarian cancer, 23–24

Cauda equina syndrome, 136
Cervical cancer
  in elderly, 13
  Pap smear abnormalities and, 141
  risk factors for, 13
  screening for, 10–13
Cervical intraepithelial neoplasia, 11, 141
Chest pain, acute non-traumatic, evaluation of, 114–117
Chest x-ray
  in acute cough, 145
  in lung cancer screening, 21
Child abuse and neglect, screening for, 33
Children
  asthma management in, 99–105
  blood pressure percentiles in
    for boys, 164
    for girls, 165
  immunization schedule for, 86–88
  obesity management in, 139
  screening in
    for abuse and neglect, 33
    for cholesterol and lipid disorders, 35
    for depression, 39
    for hearing impairment, 45–46
    for hypertension, 52
    for iron-deficient anemia, 4
    for lead poisoning, 55–56
    for liver cancer, 20
    for obesity, 57
    for thyroid disease, 64
    for visual impairment, 68
Chlamydial infection
  risk factors for, 34
  screening for, 34
Cholesterol disorders
  and heart failure, 123
  management of, 131
  screening for
    in adults, 36–37
    in children, 35
Cirrhosis, as risk factor for liver cancer, 20
Clinical breast examination (CBE), in breast cancer screening, 6–9

Cognitive impairment, screening for, 38
  instruments for, 155–156
College students, alcohol abuse screening in, 3
Colon cancer, screening for, 14–17
Colonoscopy, in colorectal cancer screening, 14–17
Colorectal cancer
  family history and, 17
  hormone replacement therapy and, 125
  risk factors for, 17
  screening for, 14–17
Colposcopy, 141
Community-acquired pneumonia, 145
Congestion, acute sinus and nasal, management of, 147
Corticosteroids
  in allergic rhinitis, 95
  in asthma, 101–103
Cough, acute, management of, 145
COX-2 inhibitors, in arthritis, 98
Cromolyn sodium
  in allergic rhinitis, 95
  in asthma, 103

D

Decongestants, in allergic rhinitis, 95
Dementia
  hormone replacement therapy and, 124
  screening for, 38
    instruments for, 155–156
Dental exam, in oral cancer screening, 22
Depression
  management of, 118
  risk factors for, 40
  screening for, 39–40
    in elderly, 157–160, 162
  suicide risk in, 39–40
Dermatitis, atopic, evaluation and management algorithm for, 106–108

Diabetes mellitus
complications of, prevention and treatment of, 120–122
gestational, screening for, 41
hypertension and, 42, 80, 120, 127
management of, 119
and myocardial infarction prevention, 80
risk factors for, 42
and stroke prevention, 91
type 2
prevention of, 74
screening for, 42
Diet
in hypertension prevention, 78
in myocardial infarction prevention, 79
in obesity management, 138–139
Digitalis, in heart failure, 123
Digital rectal exam, in prostate cancer screening, 26–27
Diphtheria-acellular pertussis-tetanus vaccine, 86
Diuretics, in hypertension, 127, 129
Domestic violence and abuse, screening for, 43
Drinking. *See* Alcohol abuse and dependence
DTaP vaccine, 86
Dual energy x-ray absorptiometry (DXA), 58

E

Ectopic pregnancy, chlamydial infection and, 34
Eczema, evaluation and management algorithm for, 106–108
Elderly
activities of daily living assessment in, 162
acute cough in, evaluation and management of, 145
fall prevention for, 76
home environment assessment for, 162
osteoporosis prevention in, 81–83

screening in
for dementia, 38
for depression, 40, 157, 159–160, 162
for domestic abuse, 43
for falls, 44, 76
for hearing impairment, 46
for hypertension, 54
for osteoporosis, 58–59
for thyroid disease, 64–65
for visual impairment, 69
Endocarditis, prevention and prophylaxis of, 75
Endometrial cancer
hormone replacement therapy and, 125
risk factors for, 18
screening for, 18
Estrogen therapy
in osteoporosis, 81, 125, 140
risks and benefits of, 124–126
Exercise
and hypertension prevention, 78
and myocardial infarction prevention, 79
Eye exams, 69, 112–113, 161

F

Falls
prevention of, 76
screening for, 44
Fasting lipids, in cholesterol and lipid screening, 35, 36
Fecal occult blood testing, in colorectal cancer screening, 14–16
Fluorescent treponemal antibody, absorbed test (FTA-ABS), 63
Fractures
osteoporotic, risk of, 60
in patients with acute lower back pain, 132
Framingham cardiac risk score instruments, 167–168
Functional assessment screening, in elderly, 161–163

G

Gastric cancer, screening for, 19
Geriatric Depression Scale, 40, 157,
   159–160
Gestational diabetes mellitus
   risk factors for, 42
   screening for, 41
Glaucoma, screening for, 68–69
Glucose tolerance test, 41
Glycogen storage disease, as risk fac-
   tor for liver cancer, 20
Government agencies, listing of,
   169–170

H

Haemophilus influenzae type B (Hib)
   vaccine, 86
Hearing impairment
   in elderly, 161
   screening for, 45–46
Heart failure
   management of, 123
Hemochromatosis, as risk factor for
   liver cancer, 20
Hepatitis A virus, vaccine for, 86, 89–90
Hepatitis B virus
   chronic infection
      as risk factor for liver cancer, 20
      screening for, 47
   vaccine for, 86, 89–90
Hepatitis C virus
   chronic infection
      as risk factor for liver cancer,
         20, 48
      screening for, 48–49
   testing algorithm for asymptomatic
      persons in, 49
Hepatocellular carcinoma
   hepatitis C and, 48
   risk factors for, 20
   screening for, 20
HIV. *See* Human immunodeficiency
   virus (HIV)
Hormone replacement therapy (HRT)
   and breast cancer, 72, 124
   in osteoporosis, 81, 125, 140
   risks and benefits of, 124–126

HRT. *See* Hormone replacement
   therapy (HRT)
Human immunodeficiency virus (HIV)
   home testing, 51
   screening for, 50–51
Human papilloma virus (HPV) infection, 11, 141
Hyperglycemia
   management of, 119
   prevention and treatment of, 74, 120
Hyperlipidemia
   and myocardial infarction preven-
      tion, 79
   prevention and treatment of, 120
   and stroke prevention, 85
   in type 2 diabetes mellitus, 42
Hypertension
   control and treatment of, 127–130
      in diabetic patients, 42, 120, 127
      and myocardial infarction, 79,
         80
      and stroke prevention, 84
   initiating therapy for, 127
   and lifestyle modifications, 78
   prevention of, 77, 78, 128
   risk factors for, 77
   screening for
      in adolescents, 52
      in adults, 53
      in children, 52
      in elderly patients, 54
   secondary causes, 54
Hypothyroidism, screening for,
   64–65

I

Immunization schedule
   for adults, 89–92
   for children, 86–88
Incontinence, functional assessment
   of, in the elderly, 161
Infants, screening in
   for hearing impairment, 45–46
   for iron-deficient anemia, 4
   for lead poisoning, 55–56
   for visual impairment, 68
Influenza vaccine, 86, 89, 90

Insulin therapy, in diabetes, 119
Isoniazid, in tuberculosis, 66

K

Kidney disease, chronic, recommended drugs for, 129

L

Lead poisoning
  risk factors for, 56
  screening for, 55–56
Leg, functional assessment of, in the elderly, 161
Lipid disorders
  in diabetic patients, 120
  management of, 131
  and myocardial infarction, 79
  risk factors for, 36–37
  screening for
    in adults, 36–37
    in children, 35
  and stroke, 85
Liver cancer, screening for, 20
Low back pain
  management of, 132–137
  red flags, 136
  surgical considerations, 135
Lung cancer, screening for, 21

M

Mammography, in breast cancer screening, 6–9
Mastectomy, in breast cancer prevention, 72, 73
Measles, mumps, rubella (MMR) vaccine, 86, 89, 90
Melanoma, 28
Men
  screening in
    for prostate cancer, 26
    for testicular cancer, 29
  10-year cardiac risk for, estimate of, 167
Meningococcal vaccine, 89, 90
Menopause, hormone replacement therapy in, 124–125

Mental status, functional assessment of, in the elderly, 162
Mild Cognitive Impairment, dementia screening in, 38
Mini Mental State Examination, 155–156
Myocardial infarction
  prevention of, 79–80
  recommended drugs for, 129

N

Nasal congestion, management of, 147
National Alcohol Screening Day, 3
Neck palpation, in thyroid cancer screening, 30
Nedocromil, in asthma, 103
Neglect, child, screening for, 33
Neonates, screening in, for iron-deficient anemia, 4
Nephropathy, diabetic, prevention and treatment of, 120
Neuropathy, diabetic, prevention and treatment of, 120
Nonsteroidal anti-inflammatory drugs (NSAIDs)
  in acute cough, 145
  in acute lower back pain, 133
  in acute rhinosinusitis, 147
  in arthritis, 98
  in sore throat, 146
Nutrition assessment, in the elderly, 161

O

Obesity
  management of
    in adults, 138
    in children, 139
  screening for, 57
Oral cancer, screening for, 22
Oral glucose tolerance test, 41
Osteoarthritis, management algorithm for, 96–98
Osteoporosis
  causes of, 61
  fracture risk in, 60

hormone replacement therapy in, 82, 124, 125, 140

managment of, 140

predictors of, 81

prevention of, 81–83

risk factors for, 60, 81

screening for, 58–59

secondary causes, 61

treatment of, 82

Osteoporosis Risk Assessment Instrument (ORAI), 58

Ovarian cancer

hormone replacement therapy and, 125

risk factors for, 24

screening for, 23–24

P

Pancreatic cancer, screening for, 25

Pap smear

abnormalities in, management and follow-up for, 141

in cervical cancer screening, 9–13

in endometrial cancer screening, 18

Pelvic exam, rectovaginal, in ovarian cancer screening, 23

Pelvic inflammatory disease, chlamydial infection and, 34

Perioperative Cardiovascular Evaluation, 142–143

Pharyngitis, management of, 146

Physical activity

in hypertension prevention, 78

in myocardial infarction prevention, 79

in type 2 diabetes prevention, 74

Pneumococcal vaccine, 86, 89–90

Pneumonia

acute cough with, 145

community-acquired, management of, 144

Polio vaccine, 86

Porphyria cutanea tarda, as risk factor for liver cancer, 20

Pregnancy, screening in

for alcohol abuse and dependence, 3

for chlamydial infection, 34

for gestational diabetes mellitus, 41

for hepatitis B infection, 47

for HIV, 51

for iron-deficient anemia, 4

for syphilis, 63

PRIME-MD (Primary Care Evaluation of Mental Disorders), for depression screening, 40, 157

Professional societies, listing of, 169–170

Progesterone/progestin therapy, risks and benefits of, 124–126

Prostate cancer

risk factors for, 27

screening for, 26–27

Prostate-specific antigen (PSA), in prostate cancer screening, 26–27

Pulmonary exam, in acute, nontraumatic chest pain, 116

R

Raloxifene

in breast cancer prevention, 73

in osteoporosis, 82, 140

Rapid plasmin reagin (RPR) test, 63

Rectal exam, in prostate cancer screening, 26–27

Renal disease, chronic, recommended drugs for, 129

Respiratory infection, upper, evaluation and management of, 146–148

Retinopathy, diabetic, prevention and treatment of, 120

Rhinitis, allergic, diagnosis and management algorithm for, 94–95

Rhinosinusitis, acute, management of, 147

Risedronate, in osteoporosis, 82, 140

S

Sciatica, persistent, surgical considerations for, 135

Scoliosis, screening for, 62
Selective estrogen receptor modulators, in osteoporosis, 82, 140
Sexually transmitted disease, screening for, 34
Sigmoidoscopy, in colorectal cancer screening, 14–17
Simple Calculated Osteoporosis Risk Estimation (SCORE), 58
Sinus congestion, management of, 147
Sinusitis, acute, management of, 147
Skin cancer
    risk factors for, 28
    screening for, 28
Smoking
    and myocardial infarction prevention, 79–80
    as risk factor for lung cancer, 21
    as risk factor for pancreatic cancer, 25
    and stroke prevention, 85
Social support, functional assessment of, in the elderly, 163
Sore throat, acute, management of, 146
Spinal stenosis, 137
Sputum cytology, in lung cancer screening, 21
Statins
    in myocardial infarction prevention, 79
    in osteoporosis prevention, 82
Steroids
    in allergic rhinitis, 95
    in asthma, 101–103
Strabismus, screening for, 68
Stroke
    hormone replacement therapy and, 125
    prevention of, 84–85
        recommended drugs for, 129
    risk factors for, 115
Suicide risk, screening for, 39–40
Syphilis, screening for, 63

T

Tamoxifen, in breast cancer prevention, 72, 73

Testicular cancer
    risk factors for, 29
    screening for, 29
Tetanus-diphtheria vaccine, 86–87
Theophylline, in asthma, 102–103
Thyroid-stimulating hormone (TSH), 64–65
Thyroid cancer, screening for, 30
Thyroid disease
    risk factors for, 65
    screening for, 64–65
Total-body skin exam, in skin cancer screening, 28
Total colon exam, in colorectal cancer screening, 16
Tuberculin skin test, 66–67
Tuberculosis, screening for, 66–67
Tyrosinemia, as risk factor for liver cancer, 20

U

Ultrasound
    in carotid artery stenosis screening, 31–32
    in heptocelllular carcinoma screening, 20
    in ovarian cancer screening, 23
    transrectal, in prostate cancer screening, 26–27
    transvaginal, in endometrial cancer screening, 18
Upper respiratory infection, evaluation and management of, 146–148
Urinary continence, functional assessment of, in the elderly, 161
Urinary tract infection, diagnosis and management algorithm for, 148–150

V

Vaccines, recommended schedules for
    for adults, 89–92
    for children, 86–88
Varicella virus vaccine, 86, 89–90

Venereal Disease Research Laboratory (VDRL) test, 63
Violence, domestic, screening for, 43
Visual impairment
  evaluation and management of, 112–113
  screening for, 68–69
    in elderly, 161
Vitamin D supplementation, in osteoporosis, 140

W

Waist-hip ratio, in obesity screening, 57
Warfarin, and stroke prevention, 90, 109–110
Weight loss
  in hypertension prevention, 78
  in myocardial infarction prevention, 79
  in obesity management, 138–139
  in type 2 diabetes prevention, 74
Weight measurements
  in body mass index conversion, 166
  in obesity screening, 57

Western blot, in HIV testing, 50
Wilson's disease, as risk factor for liver cancer, 20
Women
  breast cancer prevention in, 72–73
  osteoporosis prevention in, 81–83
  pregnant. *See* Pregnancy, screening in
  screening in
    for breast cancer, 6–9
    for cervical cancer, 9–13
    for chlamydial infection, 34
    for domestic abuse, 43
    for endometrial cancer, 18
    for iron-deficient anemia, 4
    for osteoporosis, 58–61
    for ovarian cancer, 23–24
    for thyroid disease, 64
  urinary tract infection management in, 148–150
  10-year cardiac risk for, estimate of, 168

Z

Zafirlukast, 103
Zileuton, 103